W9-CAH-670

Faith Matters
Teenagers, Religion, and Sexuality

Steve Clapp, Kristen Leverton Helbert, and Angela Zizak

Cover by Custom Maid Design

A LifeQuest Publication

Faith Matters
Teenagers, Religion, and Sexuality

Steve Clapp, Kristen Leverton Helbert, and Angela Zizak

For further information, contact: LifeQuest, 6404 S. Calhoun Street, Fort Wayne, Indiana 46807; DadofTia@aol.com; 260-744-6510.

The authors of this book are not medical professionals. While every attempt has been made to ensure the accuracy of information about topics such as contraception, HIV/AIDS, and other sexually transmitted diseases, you should always depend on a physician for counsel on medical matters.

The names and/or locations of some persons quoted in this book have been changed to protect their privacy.

Biblical quotations, unless otherwise noted, are from the New Revised Standard Version of the Bible, copyrighted 1989 by the Division of Christian Education, National Council of Churches, and are used by permission.

ISBN 1-893270-10-6

Manufactured in the United States of America

Contents

**This book is dedicated
to teenagers across the United States
who want to relate their faith
to their sexual decisions
and
to the clergy and other congregational leaders
who are seeking to help them.**

*We feel a significant debt to many people who influenced the
project on which this book is based. The project would not have
happened without the encouragement of Benita Melton. We
received especially significant guidance along the way from
Jeremy Ashworth, Doug Bauder, Debra W. Haffner, and Martin
Siegel. We have also been influenced by the work of others
in related fields including Douglas Kirby, Diane di Mauro,
and James Nelson.*

*We deeply appreciate the funding Christian Community has
received for our work in the area of youth and sexuality from
these foundations: The Compton Foundation, The Lutheran
Foundation, and The Charles Stewart Mott Foundation. Related
work has been helped by the William and Flora Hewlett Foundation, the W.T. Grant Foundation, and the Robert Sterling
Clark Foundation.*

*We extend our thanks for the contributions made to this book
by Jan Fairchild, Susan Ruth Forste, Celia King, Randy Maid,
Jerry Peterson, Stacey Sellers, Sara Sprunger, and the staff of
Evangel Press.*

So now, O Israel, what does the LORD your God require of you? Only to fear the LORD your God, to walk in all his ways, to love him, to serve the LORD your God with all your heart and with all your soul, and to keep the commandments of the LORD your God and his decrees that I am commanding you today, for your own well-being.

Deuteronomy 10:12-13

Just then a lawyer stood up to test Jesus. "Teacher," he said, "what must I do to inherit eternal life?" He said to him, "What is written in the law? What do you read there?" He answered, "You shall love the Lord your God with all your heart, and with all your soul, and with all your strength, and with all your mind; and your neighbor as yourself."

Luke 10:25-27

Chapter One
Religion, Teens, and Sex–
A Fresh Look

When I got pregnant, my minister was so kind and
helpful to me. I'll never forget how he got my parents
to stop being angry. . . . But where was the church
before I got pregnant? If I'd understood the way my
faith should shape my decisions, I don't think I
would have had intercourse. And why didn't the
church or anyone else teach me about pills or condoms?
I know what I did is my responsibility, but the right
information could have changed my life.

Female Teenager

Congregations Can Make a Difference

The teenager who shared those words is right. Her minister
came through for her in a time of tremendous need, but her
church could have helped her avoid becoming pregnant in the
first place. The good news is that things changed in that faith
community. This young woman and her pastor were responsible
for new program initiatives which started providing youth more
help in relating their faith to sexual decisions and in having the
information they need about sexuality. The whole congregation
also embraced this single parent and her daughter in ways that
enriched the two of them and the whole church.

In his classic book *Body Theology*, James Nelson points out
the problems which come when our faith communities are silent
about sexuality:

> *To the extent that our religious communities are*
> *sexually silent, we fail to bring faith's resources*
> *of support, guidance, and care to deeply significant*
> *aspects of our members' experiences. . . . Our*
> *congregations are losing countless teenagers and*
> *young adults, not to mention older persons, because*
> *they continue to be silent, timid, and negative about*
> *sexuality.*

Too many of our congregations are silent, timid, and negative about sexuality. But there are also significant signs of hope, because many clergy and other congregational leaders want to make a difference. Here are some comments from five clergy as recorded on surveys completed as part of the Teenage Sexuality and Religion Research Project:

- *You are sending this survey at a good time. We just completed a program where we trained some youth in our church so they could provide information on sexuality to their friends at school. Our teens enjoyed the study and amazed me by how frank they were about how they view sexuality. And I keep hearing the youth talking about making a difference with their friends.*

- *We had a young woman in our congregation who got pregnant last year and decided to keep the baby but not get married. That was like a wake-up call to all of us in this little church. We started asking ourselves why teens weren't getting better information about sex and birth control. The local schools don't provide it. Our parents are embarrassed to talk about it. Surely the church has responsibility in this area.*

- *I'm ashamed to say that we have done very little in this church. We participated in the 'True Love Waits' emphasis in the community, but we were critical of that program because it doesn't give teens information about their bodies or about birth control–in case they decide not to wait. They are all going to have sex eventually, and we should be helping prepare them for that and helping them see that their faith directly relates to their sexual decisions. But all we did was criticize the True Love program–we didn't do anything ourselves. As I look back, I feel good about the program, but that doesn't excuse us from doing more.*

- *Our synagogue offered a program for teenagers and their parents this year. It was the first time we've done something like this, and we were very pleased at how many took part. Some of us have been talking about the fact that youth and parents in the community could benefit from similar experiences.*

- *I will tell you straight out that I am opposed to sex ed in the public schools. It isn't because I don't want the kids to have the information. I want them to have more information than they can get in the schools, but I want it to be in the context of the teachings of the church. Who should be doing sex ed? It should be the parents and the church. And we in the church need to be equipping parents to do a better job.*

Christian Community carried out the Teenage Sexuality and Religion Research Project because we wanted to better understand how the faith and congregational activity of teenagers influence their sexual values and behaviors. Christian Community, the nonprofit organization for which we work, is continually involved in practical research about congregational life in North America. Because of our contacts with numerous local churches and other faith-based institutions over the years, we have grown increasingly concerned as individuals and as an organization because so many congregations appeared to us to be doing very little to help youth relate their faith to sexual decisions, dating, marriage, or parenting.

While the study certainly identifies some significant areas of concern and also revealed some information which surprised us, we were, on the whole, encouraged by the results–because it is so clear that large numbers of clergy and other congregational leaders want their religious communities to be doing more with sexuality education and that youth want that help from their faith-based institutions. The five clergy quotes just shared are reasonably representative of attitudes that we encountered from large number of congregational leaders across the United States.

Obviously talking with youth about some aspects of sexuality makes many clergy and other church leaders uncomfortable. It's not surprising that congregational leaders are most comfortable teaching about abstinence without any accompanying information about other aspects of sexuality. Contraception, HIV/AIDS, rape, sexual abuse, and homosexuality are more difficult topics to approach.

By the time you have finished this book, however, we think you will agree with us that the best approach is teaching abstinence as a part of comprehensive sexuality education. Young people need the help of their parents and of faith-based institutions in relating their spirituality to the many important decisions they will face during their lives as a part of dating, marriage, sexual activity, and parenting.

Even if comprehensive sexuality education through your congregation seems like a bigger step than is realistic, don't despair! First, the climate for new initiatives in this area seems to us a more positive climate than in some past periods of time. Second, *any* new actions in helping youth relate their faith to their decisions about sexuality can make a positive difference.

According to Gallup, Search Institute, and the Kaiser Family Foundation, over 90% of the teenagers in the United States self-identify as religious, and around 60% of them spend time in a church or synagogue. Faith-based institutions have the opportunity to have tremendous influence on young people. There are several reasons why we feel it is important for faith-based institutions to undertake initiatives in sexuality education:

1. Because churches and other faith-based institutions have a deep concern about young people and their development, we have an obligation to provide them with the information and the guidance that they need in this area of life. When young people do not receive the information that they need, early sexual activity, teen pregnancy, HIV/AIDS, other sexually transmitted diseases, rape, and sexual abuse can all be a result. Young people pay a price when those of us in the religious community fail to take seriously our responsibility to them.

2. Because decisions about dating, marriage, sexual activity, and parenting are moral and spiritual decisions, parents and religious institutions are the ones with the responsibility for imparting the beliefs, values, and information to shape those decisions. While there are important reasons for having sexuality education available through the public schools, it is not the job of public schools to impart the spiritual foundation that those of us in the religious community can offer young people in their decision-making.

3. Evidence exists from secular studies that short term efforts at sexuality education are helpful but that many other factors are involved in helping lower early sexual activity by teens, reduce teen pregnancy rates, and lower instances of HIV/AIDS and other sexually transmitted diseases. How young

people feel about themselves, how successful they are in school, and how connected they are with their family and significant adults can all have an impact on how early they commence sexual activity.   In *No Easy Answers*, an excellent publication from the National Campaign to Prevent Teen Pregnancy, Douglas Kirby writes that for more impact, programs "need to effectively address a greater number of risk and protective factors over a long period of time" [p. 1].

Because churches and other faith-based institutions relate to children and their parents from the time of birth, there are numerous opportunities to help guide the development of young people in positive ways.   Service projects and other experiences which help build the self-esteem of youth are a routine part of the life of many congregations.   If age-appropriate sexuality education is added to the many other positive experiences congregations make possible for youth, the potential exists for significant impact on their lives.

4.   The teachings of the Christian, Jewish, Muslim, Hindu, and Buddhist traditions include an emphasis on reaching out to people who are in need.   The values of compassion, generosity, hospitality, and concern are common to all the major faith traditions.   Teen pregnancy, HIV/AIDS, and poverty are realities which people of faith would like to reduce.   Churches and other faith-based institutions can help not only their own young people but also young people in the community.   With congregations in every neighborhood in the United States, there is tremendous potential for positive impact on these social problems if faith-based institutions can identify effective strategies.

5.   Some persons, who are uncomfortable with any institution offering sexuality education to young people, feel that parents are the ones who should provide this information. Churches and other faith-based institutions already have the involvement of both children and parents. They are in an ideal position to provide the guidance to parents that is needed if they are to be sexuality educators to their children.   Our own bias is that congregations should both provide guidance to parents in this important area and also provide sexuality education directly to youth.   If the direct provision of that education to youth by the congregation isn't considered appropriate, then the provision of guidance to parents becomes even more crucial.

6. Congregational activities not only foster close relationships among young people who participate but also between young people and the adults who serve as their teachers, youth group advisors, and clergy. Those relationships have the potential to tremendously impact the moral development of young people. We need to create an atmosphere in our faith-based institutions in which youth can comfortably talk with each other and with adults about sexuality, dating, marriage, and parenting.

Our faith-based institutions really are in a unique position to make a very positive difference in the lives of young people, including those in the community as well as those already active in congregational life. Our hope is that the pages of this book will not only help you understand why it is so important for your congregation to help youth in these areas but will also provide you with specific strategies which can be used in your congregation or other faith-based institution.

We began the Teenage Sexuality and Religion Research Project with some important questions we wanted to investigate. Some of the results were what we expected, but others surprised us. As you read the pages which follow, we encourage you to do so with an open mind. Some of the information may shock you, and some of it may be difficult to accept. But the overall news is good–our faith-based institutions can make a difference in the lives of our young people. A better understanding of how the religious beliefs and congregational activity of teens influence their sexual values and behaviors is a good starting point. Then we must decide how to respond.

Sexuality–Not Isolated from the Rest of Teenage Life

In "Sexuality Research in the United States," Diane di Mauro reminds us that "much sexual research focuses on sexuality as represented by risk behaviors. By this very definition, sexuality is negatively viewed as the source of problems and disease rather than as an integral part of human development and health. . . . What we know about adolescent sexuality is what the literature on teenage pregnancy and HIV/AIDS tells us" [*Researching Sexual Behavior*, edited by John Bancroft, p. 3].

While much of the information shared in *Faith Matters* focuses on risk behaviors, we designed the Teenage Sexuality and Religion Research Project to learn as much as possible about the overall way in which youth view sexuality–in relationship to their spiritual lives, their relationships with other youth and adults, their thinking about and planning for marriage and parenting, and other factors in their lives. If those of us who embrace religious faith truly accept the view that sexuality is a good gift from a loving God, it is important to know to what extent that perspective is being communicated to our youth.

When many of us hear the word sexuality, our minds go to those parts of the body known as genitals and to the activities which people do using those body parts. Most of us know that sexuality is more than that, but we don't often think about the implications of that reality. There are many excellent definitions of sexuality, but we have become partial to one shared by James B. Nelson in *Between Two Gardens*:

> *By sexuality I mean not only physiological arousal and genital activity, but also much more. While human sexuality is not the whole of our personhood, it is a basic dimension of that personhood. While it does not determine all thought, feelings, and action, it does permeate and affect all of these. Sexuality is our way of being in the world as male and female.* [p. 5]

Another good definition comes from the Surgeon General of the United States (2001):

> *We must understand that sexuality encompasses more than sexual behavior, that the many aspects of sexuality include not only the physical, but the mental and spiritual as well, and that sexuality is a core component of personality. . . Sexual health is not limited to the absence of disease or dysfunction, nor is its importance confined to just the reproductive years. It includes the ability to understand and weigh the risks, responsibilities, outcomes, and impacts of sexual action and to practice abstinence when appropriate. It includes freedom from sexual abuse and discrimination and the ability of individuals to integrate their sexuality into their lives, derive pleasure from it, and to reproduce if they so choose.*

When we focus our efforts at helping youth only on the prevention of pregnancy and of HIV/AIDS and other sexually transmitted diseases, we fail to do what we should to help them understand themselves as sexual beings and to prepare them for the sexual relationships which will be part of their lives. A very frank Lutheran pastor with whom we visited suggested to us with humor what has too often been the truth of what we have taught youth: "Sex is something dirty and unpleasant. Save it for the one you love." (Sexuality educator Sol Gordon shared similar words in his books and speeches. The quote may have originated with him.)

As you read the pages which follow, you'll discover that many youth feel they have received little information about sexuality from their faith-based institutions except prohibitions and that too much sexuality education has been primarily fear-based. We can do better, and we can help teens better understand how their spirituality should inform their understanding of their sexuality.

If we accept Nelson's view that sexuality is our way of being in the world as male and female, then we need to provide youth with the full information they need to relate their spirituality to their sexuality. We need to be preparing them not only for sexual decisions but also for dating, for marriage, and for the time when they themselves will be parents. Many of our congregations are alarmed by high divorce rates, but we often miss opportunities to help youth have the knowledge and guidance which will help them make healthy choices of marriage partners, build solid marriage relationships, and keep their wedding vows.

We are also increasingly aware of the reality that not all young people seek heterosexual relationships. Some will determine that they are homosexual or bisexual in orientation and will be in a homosexual relationship. Many of our religious communities are divided over this issue, with some people feeling that homosexual behavior is sinful and with others feeling that it is a part of God's design and should be as affirmed as heterosexual behavior.

All of our faith-based institutions face a tremendous challenge in deciding how to relate to teens who have a homosexual orientation or who have questions about their orientation. Whatever your personal beliefs on this potentially divisive topic in congregational life, we urge you to remember as you read the results of our study and as you relate to youth that those of homosexual orientation remain the children of God.

Studying Youth, Religion, and Sexuality

The study reported in the pages of this book is certainly not the first or the last to deal with the relationship among youth, religion, and sexuality. When we first sketched what we wanted to report at the end of this project, we intended to include at least a substantial appendix which shared what some others have done in this area. This task, however, has already been done for us in the National Campaign to Prevent Teen Pregnancy publication *Keeping the Faith: The Role of Religion and Faith Communities in Preventing Teen Pregnancy* by Barbara Dafoe Whitehead, Brian L. Wilcox, and Sharon Scales Rostosky. Those interested in such an overview of research by others will find considerable help in that publication.

With many other studies looking at teen sexual behavior, why did we feel it was important to do one more? We think that question warrants an answer. Here are some of the factors that we felt were important in the design of this study:

1. As shared in the earlier quote from Diane di Mauro, much of the study of sexuality done in the United States is focused on risk behaviors. Research is expensive, and there is an understandable tendency for projects to be funded primarily because they address some significant problem such as teen pregnancy or HIV/AIDS. Our study certainly looked carefully at risk behaviors, but we designed it to learn as much as possible about the overall way in which youth view sexuality.

2. Many studies on teen sexual attitudes and behavior examine religious variables, but religion is not the major focus. Often "religion is tangential to the main focus of these studies and is used to statistically control for its potential effect on the relationship between the main variables of interest and sexual behavior" [*Keeping the Faith*, p. 37]. It's common in such studies for the religious affiliation of teens to simply be identified as Protestant, Catholic, or "other." Those categories are very broad given the diversity of teachings in many religious traditions. It's

15

also common in such studies to look at worship attendance or another single variable to measure how religious teens are. From the beginning of our study, religious beliefs and congregational activity were our primary focuses of interest. We sought information on a large number of religious variables and wanted to understand the full range of the relationship of teens with their congregations–including how they feel about adult teachers and leaders, clergy, and other participating teens.

3. Some of the studies which have been conducted that looked more closely at religious variables have been relatively small in size and have looked at teenagers alone. Our study involved 635 congregations with 5,819 teenagers (grades nine through twelve), 635 clergy, and 442 adult youth workers completing surveys. We also conducted focus groups and interviews involving large numbers of teens, clergy, youth workers, and parents. Because the clergy responses were so interesting, we conducted a supplemental clergy survey to enlarge that portion of our database from 635 to 2,049.

4. We designed this study to look closely at what religious communities were and were not doing to help youth relate their faith to sexual decisions, dating, marriage, and parenting. We wanted to gain a better understanding of what approaches were proving most effective. Our target audience for the results of the study, from the beginning, was not family planning professionals, sexuality educators, or sexuality researchers–though we hope those persons will find our results of interest. Our target audience consists of clergy, adult teachers and leaders of youth in congregational settings, parents for whom religious faith is important, and youth who are active in their congregations.

Sociology, sexuality education, theology, and religious institutions all have their own jargon. While we have attempted to minimize the amount of that jargon in this book, it is impossible to eliminate all of it. There will be places where professionals in all these fields will wish we had been more precise in our use of terminology. Our goal has been to provide a book which will, we hope, be easy to read by persons from a variety of backgrounds including teenagers and their parents.

Research Changes Its Own Results

In *The Invisible Touch*, Harry Beckwith reminds us that "research changes its own results" [p. 7]. No matter how large the sample or how meticulous the research, there are many variables which cannot be controlled; and the research instruments and methods influence the results–sometimes in unanticipated ways. As you read this book and think about the information we are sharing, please keep in mind:

1. The youth who participated in the written surveys, interviews, and focus groups were all reached through faith-based institutions. That was an intentional part of the design because we wanted to study youth who were highly involved in congregational life. The fact that youth were reached in that way and that many surveys were completed in youth classes and groups in those institutions certainly affects the results. The process used was designed to protect confidentiality: no names or codes were put on the surveys; youth were asked but not required to identify their congregations; youth sealed their own surveys in response envelopes; and youth put their surveys in the mail rather than handing them to an adult.

It's still possible, however, that youth did not feel free to be completely candid in their responses in some settings. Would youth, for example, be as willing to admit having had sexual intercourse on this survey as they would have in a secular setting?

2. Because we intentionally wanted youth who were active in faith-based institutions, our sample is not a random one. The youth we reached are very involved in their congregations. That constitutes both a strength and a weakness of this study.

What would the results look like had the study been done on a truly random sample of youth in the United States? What differences might be observed among youth who are highly active in their congregations, youth who are only moderately active, and those who have no congregational affiliation? While we were careful in the wording of many survey items to permit comparisons with the results of some secular studies, those comparisons are risky because the studies have been done at different points in time and in different settings.

In comparing the levels of sexual activity shared in this study with the levels of activity from secular samples, it is important to remember that this data is from the year 2000. Many of the recently published reports on secular samples are from 1995, 1996, and 1997; and five or six years is a long time in terms of the changing youth culture.

Likewise, in looking at the data in this book, it is important to remember that the figures shared are the result of bivariate analysis or cross-tabulation of the variables studied. The information provided is by association but is not necessarily causal. For those not familiar with statistical methodology, a classic analogy is that the population of storks in a given geographical area may increase at the same time as the birth rate increases for that area–but this does not prove that storks bring babies.

3. The size of the sample decreases with year in school and age. There were more 9th graders than 10th graders, more 10th graders than 11th graders, and more 11th graders than 12th graders. That is consistent with the typical attendance patterns of youth in faith-based institutions.

Are those who drop out of activity in a faith-based institution more sexually active than those who continue to be involved? This makes it difficult to interpret some of the data. For example, the pregnancy rates of teens participating in this study were lower than those in some secular studies. We certainly hope that the fact these teens are strongly involved in their congregations is at least part of the reason for that difference. We need to recognize, however, that some youth who are more sexually active may decide to drop out of congregational life; and it's also possible that some teens who became pregnant decided to drop out of congregational activity at that time or were actually required to leave.

4. Faith-based institutions which agreed to participate in this study are likely to be more progressive in their willingness to deal with sexual issues than faith-based institutions which chose not to participate. Clergy and sometimes other congregational leaders had to consent to the study, and parents had to be willing for their children to participate.

We used commercial lists of faith-based institutions and used a random methodology to select congregations for an invitation to participate in the study. Overall, 24% of those invited to participate chose to do so. Some additional invitations were given to provide better ethnic and geographic diversity. The commercial lists which were utilized are likely to have underrepresented small congregations which don't have listed telephones or aren't included in official denominational directories. The sample did include a broad range of congregations in terms of the theological spectrum, including some which would be considered fundamentalist–but a fundamentalist congregation willing to take part in this study may differ in some significant ways from one which declined to do so.

About the Sample

As already shared, surveys were returned by 5,819 youth in grades nine through twelve from 635 congregations. Most surveys were completed in the fall of 2000. Slightly more females (3,070) than males (2,739) completed surveys, which is consistent with the fact that most Protestant and Catholic congregations in the United States have slightly more female teenagers than male teenagers involved.

Respondents by Religious Affiliation

4,198	Protestant
819	Roman Catholic
131	Unitarian
361	Jewish
207	Islamic
103	Other

Surveys were completed by 4,198 Protestant youth who came from 38 different denominations, including those that would be described as mainline, evangelical, conservative, and fundamentalist. Surveys were also completed by 819 Roman Catholic youth. The 361 Jewish youth completing surveys came from both Reformed and Conservative congregations, but none were from Orthodox Jewish congregations.

For the purposes of this study, we considered those in the Anabaptist tradition (Church of the Brethren, Mennonite, Brethren Church, Brethren in Christ) as part of the broader Protestant category because of the similarity in beliefs. Surveys were returned by 207 Islamic youth. There were surveys from 103 youth whom we classified as "other" in terms of religious affiliation; those included youth in the Buddhist and Hindu traditions as well as some youth who are in what might be called "new age" faith communities.

Some readers will be interested in the denominations included under the broad category of "Protestant." They are listed here in order of youth surveys received beginning with the United Methodist Church, from which we received the most surveys, and ending with the Primitive Baptist Church, from which we received the smallest number of surveys:

United Methodist Church
Presbyterian Church, USA
Southern Baptist Churches
Missouri Synod Lutheran
Evangelical Lutheran Church
African Methodist Episcopal
United Church of Christ
Disciples of Christ
American Baptist Churches
African Methodist Episcopal Zion
Episcopal Church
Assemblies of God
Church of God
Nazarene Church
Black Baptist Church
Christian Methodist Episcopal
Missionary Church
Independent Christian Churches
Pentecostal Church
Cumberland Presbyterian Church

Church of the Brethren
Mennonite Church
Pentecostal Holiness Church
Reformed Church in America
Free Methodist Church
Progressive Baptist Church
Church of Jesus Christ of
  Latter Day Saints
Evangelical Covenant Church
Friends
United Pentecostal Church
National Primitive Baptist
Moravian Church
Brethren Church
Brethren in Christ Church
Independent Baptist Church
Missionary Alliance Church
Wesleyan Church
Primitive Baptist Church

Two-thirds of the youth who completed surveys are white, but the other third includes African American, Hispanic/Latino, Native American, and Asian youth. Most of the congregations participating in the study were not multicultural to any significant extent. All but 61 of the African American youth, for example, were from congregations which were over 90% African American. Roman Catholic parishes reflected slightly greater ethnic diversity than the typical Protestant congregation which participated in the study.

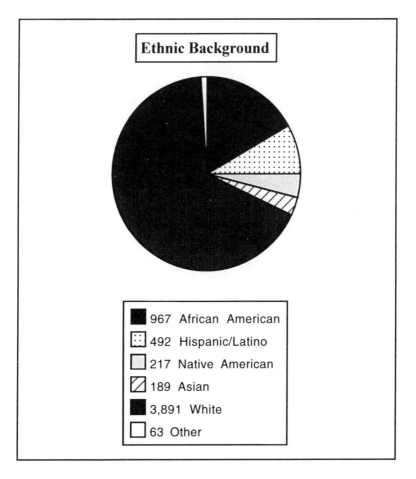

Every state was represented except New Hampshire and Utah. A few Canadian churches learned of the study and asked to participate in the survey process. While we were pleased to share the surveys with those congregations, the results were not included both because the focus was on the United States and because all the United States congregations were ones whose participation we requested based on a carefully developed sampling process rather than ones which approached us.

The teens came from a broad range of economic levels and every conceivable living arrangement including traditional husband-and-wife households, single parent homes, non-married couple households, foster homes, and households headed by couples of the same sex. Some lived with their grandparents or in the home of a friend rather than with their own parents, and some were living in children's homes or other institutional settings. A few were married, and a few were parents.

As shared earlier, there were more freshmen than sophomores, more sophomores than juniors, and more juniors than seniors completing surveys:

Year in School

1,236	12th Grade
1,363	11th Grade
1,581	10th Grade
1,639	9th Grade

The youth in this study are all active in congregational life. Not all of them attend worship services every single week, but their overall frequency of attendance is high, as indicated below. Over 80% of teens in this study attended religious services at least two or three times a month.

Attendance at Religious Services

53.8%	Attend religious services one or more times a week
26.9%	Attend religious services two or three times a month
9.5%	Attend religious services once a month
7.1%	Attend religious services less than once a month
2.7%	Never attend religious services

Activity in a youth group, youth class, choir, or other church program was higher than attendance at religious services for the youth in this study. Over 90% participate in a youth group, class, choir, or other congregational program at least two or three times a month. Those youth in our study who do not attend religious services were nevertheless active in other aspects of congregational life–especially in a youth class or group.

Frequency of Participation in Other Congregational Activities

65.3%   Participate in a youth group, youth class, choir, or other congregational program other than religious services at least once a week.

26.6%   Participate in a youth group, youth class, choir, or other congregational program other than religious services two or three times a month

4.6%   Participate in a youth group, youth class, choir, or other congregational program other than religious services once a month.

2.2%   Participate in a youth group, youth class, choir, or other congregational program other than religious services less than once a month.

1.3%   Do not participate in any congregational program other than religious services.

We found that 70.8% of the youth responding participate in two or more activities in addition to religious services. Even some of the youth who acknowledge that their frequency of participation is less than once a month nevertheless consider themselves to be part of more than one congregational group. Protestant youth were more likely than youth in other traditions to be involved in two or more activities in addition to religious services. Many Protestant youth participate in a class on Sunday morning in addition to a youth group which meets during the evening.

The smaller the congregation in our study, the more likely that youth would participate in multiple activities, if those opportunities were available. Some small congregations are not able to offer activities just for youth, though many youth in those congregations still participate in a class with adults or with younger children. Some large congregations offer an enormous range of activities for youth including sports groups, drama groups, Bible study groups, prayer groups, personal growth groups, film-making groups, and a variety of musical groups. There are youth who attend weekly Bible study groups that meet at six o'clock in the morning!

Sixty-two percent of the youth had been involved in some kind of service project through their faith-based institution. Those projects ranged from doing yard clean-up for elderly members of the congregation to traveling to other countries to help build or renovate housing for the poor. Sixteen percent of the youth in this study have helped build a Habitat for Humanity home in the United States, working with others in their congregation.

Faith is very important in the lives of almost all of these teens. Most of the teens say that they pray daily or at least weekly (95.3%), and most feel that their faith does relate to the decisions they make in their daily lives (90.2%). We asked the teens about the importance of faith in their lives: 70.5% said faith is very important in their lives, and 23.3% said it is fairly important. These responses are illustrated in the chart on the next page.

Here are some statements from teens about their faith and about congregational life:

My faith is the most important thing in the world to me. . . . The church matters more to me than school or sports or television or anything else. My mother almost died from cancer two years ago. The church was really there for my family. I can't tell you how many times the pastor and people in the congregation came to see us and prayed for us and even brought meals to us. They made the faith come alive. Female–United Methodist Church

I had been turned off on the church for years. But I started getting active in Youth for Christ, and in time I started going to church again with a friend from that group. I've turned my life over to Christ, and it's changed everything. I still screw up, but I'm becoming a better person. My temper's too short, and my mouth's too big, but I keep doing better with the help of Jesus. Male–Nondenominational Church

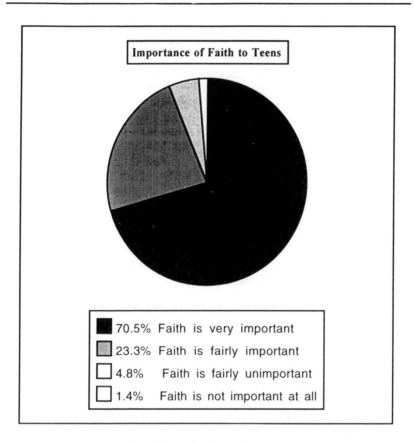

Importance of Faith to Teens

- 70.5% Faith is very important
- 23.3% Faith is fairly important
- 4.8% Faith is fairly unimportant
- 1.4% Faith is not important at all

I grew up in the church, and Christ has always been important in my family. I can't remember a time that I didn't believe in God. Male–Mennonite Church

I used to think of being Jewish as more of a cultural thing than a religious thing. My parents aren't all that religious, but they wanted me to go to Hebrew School. We have this wonderful rabbi and great instructor, and they changed my life. I see God as the center of my life now. And I think that the way faith has become so important to me has made a difference in the lives of my parents. We talk about things we never did before. Female–Synagogue (Reformed)
I got in such an awful depression that I was ready to kill myself. I was sitting in the car in the garage, with

*the door shut, and I was ready to turn the car on. My
Mom would have found me in the morning. But as I was
starting to turn the key, it's like I heard this voice speaking
to me in my head. It told me that I was loved and that God
wanted me to serve him with my life. It scared the crap
out of me. I couldn't go ahead and start the car.* Male–
Assembly of God

*The youth group in this church is where all my real
friends are. I feel a little strange sometimes because
I'm not as sure about my faith as the others in the group.
Why did Jesus have to die for us to be saved? Why
would God require that if God is so loving? Would a God
who loves us condemn all the Jews and Buddhists to hell?
The church is important to me, but I can't buy the whole
package.* Female–African Methodist Episcopal

*Even before my first communion, the Church was very
important to me. I attended our parish school until I was
ready to start high school, and that helped me. The
teachers were all religious, and they helped us see that
faith was a part of everything that we do. I'm glad to be
in a public school now, but I'll always be thankful for
St. John's.* Female–Roman Catholic

*Sometimes friends who aren't Muslim will make fun of
me because I keep halal. That means there are some
things like pork that I don't eat. I know that the pork
won't "hurt" me. . . . It's important to have some rituals
that remind you of who you are and of what's important
in your life. Not eating pork is also a way of my saying
to others that belief matters more than popularity.* Female–
Muslim

Here are a few comments from teens about the process of
taking the survey and about the link between their faith and
their sexuality:

When our rabbi asked us to do this [take the survey], *we
thought it was a scream. . . . Then we started talking about
why we don't talk about sex. There's this gap between our
faith and our hooking up with someone. We need to be
learning more about what God expects. The rabbi agrees.*
Male–Synagogue (Conservative)

I was like in shock when this survey was given to the youth group. We NEVER talk about any of this. People totally think this doesn't belong in the church. But we'll have some interesting talk after we've sealed these in the envelopes. Male–Southern Baptist Church

My minister and youth advisor encourage us to talk about sex. That's helped me sort out what I believe and how I want to live. . . But this survey makes me realize there are some topics we haven't covered yet. Female–United Church of Christ

I'm sure glad we seal these in envelopes and put them in the mail rather than handing them in. I could never have been honest if there was any chance that my teacher or pastor would find out what I had done or what I thought. Male–Church of God

This is the one topic we never touch. The only thing the church wants to say about sex is DON'T DO IT. But that isn't enough. Filling this out makes me think there must be some churches that are doing more. Are there? Female–Evangelical Lutheran Church

My priest, the church, my parents would consider me a slut if they knew what I did. . . . I don't think I'm that different than any other teenager. I can't wait to see the results of this. Like I take my religion seriously, but I can't agree with NO birth control, NO premarital sex, NO abortion under any circumstances. Female– Roman Catholic Church

Did I waste my time answering these questions? I hope not. Jesus is so important to me, and my best buds are in the youth group. . . . I want so much to do what Jesus wants with my body, but it's so hard. All my friends need so much more help than the church gives us. Female– United Pentecostal Church

27

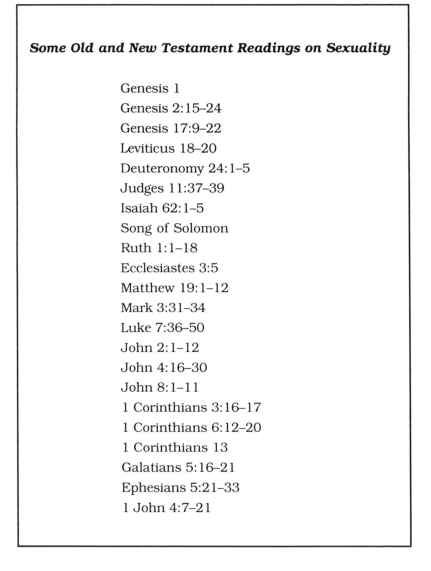

Some Old and New Testament Readings on Sexuality

Genesis 1
Genesis 2:15–24
Genesis 17:9–22
Leviticus 18–20
Deuteronomy 24:1–5
Judges 11:37–39
Isaiah 62:1–5
Song of Solomon
Ruth 1:1–18
Ecclesiastes 3:5
Matthew 19:1–12
Mark 3:31–34
Luke 7:36–50
John 2:1–12
John 4:16–30
John 8:1–11
1 Corinthians 3:16–17
1 Corinthians 6:12–20
1 Corinthians 13
Galatians 5:16–21
Ephesians 5:21–33
1 John 4:7–21

Chapter Two
Sexuality Is More than Sex

*I know this isn't completely fair, but I sometimes
think all guys want is to get you to have sex. It's
like they don't even recognize you as a whole person.
But my mother taught me that the brain is the most
important sex organ. If a guy isn't interested in what's
between my ears, he's never going to put a hand
below my waist.*

Female Teenager

Sexuality Is More than Sex

Both adults and teens can fall into the trap of thinking that
sexuality is nothing more than the act of intercourse. Consider
these comments:

*I agree that the church needs to help kids know how to
handle sex, but I don't see that as a complicated thing.
Having sexual intercourse before you're married is a sin.
We need to teach that. Teens need to know that they
should say NO.* Adult Youth Group Advisor–Church
of God

*What is the big deal about sex? You put your penis
into the girl, and both of you have a good time. Why
does everybody get so worked up about it–like it was
this big thing?* Male–Southern Baptist Church

While the adult youth advisor wants teens to know that
sexual intercourse is wrong before marriage and the teenager
sees nothing wrong with casual sex, sexuality for both of them
appears to mean nothing more than intercourse. Sexuality, as
discussed in the last chapter, really involves the whole way in
which we relate to the world as males and females. Reducing the
focus of our thinking from sexuality to sexual intercourse can
cause us to:

- Miss the reality that how we feel about ourselves, our
  relationships, and our bodies is part of our sexuality–
  and how we care for our bodies is part of our sexuality.

- Miss the importance of relationships in healthy sexuality. We are sexual beings in the midst of all our relationships–not just when dating or engaging in sexual behaviors.

- Forget that there are many forms of sexual activity in addition to intercourse. Masturbation, kissing, flirting, and massaging are all sexual behaviors, as are petting and oral sex.

- Miss the reality that there is a spiritual dimension to sexuality which goes beyond the prohibition of certain behaviors and includes recognizing that sexuality is one of God's gifts!

Feelings about the Body

The Jewish and Christian faiths teach that we are created in the image of God, and the Old and New Testaments speak of the value of the body. Our feelings about our bodies and the bodies of others are part of our sexuality. We live in a culture which promotes certain body images through advertising, television shows, motion pictures, and the Internet. Thin women and well-muscled men are the norm in the entertainment industry, and most ordinary people don't meet those standards of attractiveness.

We asked the teens in this study to choose from one of four options to describe how happy they were with their bodies. The chart on the next page shows the responses from the young people, and you can see significant differences between the way that teenage males and teenage females feel about their bodies. Among the females in this study, 61.9% were somewhat or definitely unhappy with their bodies; 19.5% were happy but still wanted some improvement; and only 18.6% were happy without qualification. The comparable figures for males were 48.5% somewhat or definitely unhappy; 17.2% happy but wanting some improvement, and 24.3% happy without qualification. Almost twice as many girls as boys were "definitely unhappy" with their bodies. Still, many boys are unhappy and want changes.

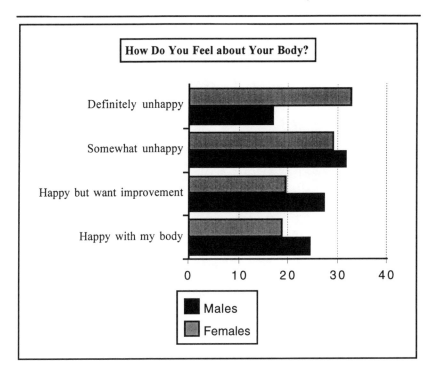

How Do You Feel about Your Body?

Some of the teens had very strong feelings about their appearance and the importance that attractiveness played in their lives:

I hate my body. I diet, I exercise, I do everything right. But it doesn't make any difference. I still have ten pounds that won't go away, and that keeps me from looking like I should. . . . Two of my friends have bigger weight problems than I do and think I shouldn't complain. But I don't want to look like this. Female–Missouri Synod Lutheran

White people are the ones with the problem about weight. Black people aren't as concerned. We look more at what's in a person's heart. This is one of the differences between the races. I get so ripped because my white girlfriends are always worried about their weight and their muscles. Get a life, people. Female–Roman Catholic Church

31

---

*I was a fat baby, and I'm a fat high school student. I'm
smart. I'm funny. I know lots of girls who like to be
with me and ask my opinions. They wouldn't go on
a date with me though. I don't look good enough. They
have to see themselves as being able to get someone better
than me to ask them out.* Male–Southern Baptist Church

*I had a birthmark on my face until three years ago. Then
a plastic surgeon used this new method to help me grow
a balloon of skin on the side of my face. I went into hiding
for the summer while the skin was growing. Then he
used my own skin to fix the birthmark. The difference was
awesome. I look so good now, and it feels so good. But
I know who my real friends are. My real friends are the
ones who liked me before the surgery. These guys who
wouldn't give me a second look before the surgery, I have
no second look for them now. In one way I'm so happy
with how I look, but in another I'm not. When I had
the ugly blotch on my face, it was easy to know who
cared about the real me, the me that no one sees on the
surface.* Female–Presbyterian Church U.S.A.

*I looked like such a dork in middle school. Now I've grown
more, and I've been lifting weights and running. My sister
says I look like a hunk. She's like drop dead beautiful, so
I guess she should know, but I still don't see myself that
way. I keep thinking I must look like a dork. I have this
low self-confidence in talking to girls that I can't seem to
get past.* Male–Synagogue (Conservative)

*I worry about my sister so much. She was a little heavy
until the summer of her freshman year. Then she went
on this diet and started running every day. She looks so
hot now. That should be a good thing, but down inside
she still sees herself as pudgy. She wants affection from
guys so much that she'll do almost anything to get it.
She doesn't have enough pride in herself, and she has the
rep of being "easy." It makes me feel so bad for her.
Appearance has so much to do with everything.* Male–
Friends Meeting

*I know the Bible teaches that we were made in the image
of God. Well, if I'm in that image, then I guess God's pretty
average because that's what I am. I look okay, but I'm*

never going to be the one that boys turn in the hall to stare at. . . . I wouldn't want to be like a couple of my friends who will do anything to keep their weight down. My friend Beth has an eating disorder. I'm so worried about her and even had my mother talk to her mother about it. I have another friend who doesn't have an eating disorder, but she's so careful about everything that goes into her mouth. That's no way to live. . . . It wouldn't be a problem except for my wanting some great looking guy to take an interest in me. Why do I want that? I feel good about myself, and I'm average. Why can't I feel okay about a guy who's average? Female–Evangelical Covenant Church

I don't think appearance is as important to women as it is to men. But there are some basics. There's this guy that I used to go out with who had skanky breath most of the time. I'd hold my breath to kiss him so I didn't gag. I finally told him about it, and I hurt his feelings so much that he cried. I was so sorry, but I thought he ought to know. Female–Church of Jesus Christ of Latter Day Saints

The African American teens in the sample were more likely than the other ethnic groups to feel good about their physical appearance. The female quoted on page 31 is not the only black person in the study to express frustration with the emphasis that white people put on weight and appearance.

Seventy-seven percent of the females and 39% of the males in the study have been on a diet sometime in the last year. The figures for African Americans were lower but are still high (55% of females and 27% for males). Six percent of the females and 1.5% of the males acknowledge that they have or have had an eating disorder. This was a request for self-identification, so the actual number may be higher. Almost all the teens of both sexes acknowledge that they know someone with an eating disorder.

We asked the teens to rate the importance of physical attractiveness and seven other characteristics in determining whether or not to date or go out with a person. There were some definite male and female differences, and those changed with year in school. A characteristic marked "one" would be the most important; one marked "eight" would be the least important. This table shows the average rank given to appearance:

Ranking of Appearance from Eight Characteristics In Deciding to Date or Go Out with a Person

	Males	**Females**
Freshmen	Five	Four
Sophomores	Four	Four
Juniors	Three	Five
Seniors	Two	Six

The older females placed less importance on physical appearance than the younger females in contrast to the older males who placed more importance on appearance than the younger males. In any exercise like this, there is the possibility, of course, that some teens were answering as they felt they *should* rather than as actually do feel.

In talking with groups of teens about the results of the study, we've raised the question of why older females seem to put so much less importance than males on appearance in deciding whether or not to date or go out with a person. A female senior shared this perspective, which was echoed by several others:

This culture evaluates women so much by the way they look. The older you grow, the more you realize just how true this is and how unfair it is. You are so much more than your appearance, and it is so wrong for society to make looks so important. I think that causes a girl, a woman not to want to use the same standards toward men that are used toward them. But then there's also the problem of being honest with yourself about this.

When asked to predict how much importance the opposite sex put on each characteristic, both males and females, with the exception of one category, thought the other sex would rank physical attractiveness higher than they actually did. The exception came with senior girls who felt, on average, that males their age would give attractiveness a ranking of three rather than two. In talking about the results, some female teenagers have expressed anger over the importance that males put on appearance in deciding to date or go out with someone:

34

*I find this really disappointing. These are church active,
religious guys. And the older they get, the more important
they think appearance is. How shallow. It makes me think
that I don't want to go out with anyone.* Female–junior

*I believe these statistics. Absolutely. I have these two
terrific friends who are both just a little overweight. They
both, to me, look attractive and are so smart and so nice.
They hardly ever get asked out. I tried fixing one of them
up for the prom, and the appearance thing was it with
all three of the fellows I approached. Damn. You would
think that people who were involved in the church would
have different responses. You'd think they'd be trying to
see other people as God sees us.* Female–senior

The females weren't the only ones disappointed. Some of the
males who saw the results were not happy with their male
friends. For example:

*This makes me feel ashamed. Why are guys so narrow-
minded? Some of us need to do some serious praying about
this. It feels like a sin to be judging other people so much
on the basis of appearance.* Male–junior

Sexual Intercourse

The youth completing our surveys show lower rates of sexual
intercourse than is reflected in most secular studies. The rates
are lower for all the subgroups we have analyzed in the survey
including Caucasian teens, African American teens, Hispanic
teens, evangelical teens, Catholic teens, mainline Protestant
teens, Unitarian Universalist teens, Jewish teens, and Muslim
teens.

Several participants in the focus groups we held in the
process of designing the study predicted that it would show
lower rates of sexual intercourse among youth from evangelical
or fundamentalist denominations than among youth from
mainline Protestant or Roman Catholic traditions. That was not
the case. No particular religious traditions showed markedly
lower rates of sexual intercourse than other religious traditions
except for Jewish and Muslim youth, who were less likely to have
had intercourse than Christian youth.

We did, however, find a subcategory of teens who had rates of sexual intercourse which were not only lower than many secular studies have shown but which were also lower than for the other teens in this study. Those teens (1,093 or 18.8%) share these characteristics:

- They attend religious services one or more times a week.
- They pray daily.
- They have involvement in at least one congregational group besides religious education and worship.
- They say that the teachings of the congregation and/or the Scriptures have "a lot of influence" on their sexual decisions.
- They say the congregation has provided information on how to make sexual decisions and on what the Scriptures says about sexuality.
- They feel a strong connection with congregational leaders who work with youth.
- They feel a strong connection with other youth in the congregation.
- They feel the adults who work with them portray sex in a healthy and positive way.
- They say their congregation encourages abstinence from intercourse for high school aged people.

The encouragement of abstinence is a factor, but it is only one factor in this group of youth who were especially unlikely to have had intercourse. Most of the factors are positive in nature: strong attendance and involvement in the faith community, strong connections with other youth and with adults who work with youth, and what they see as a healthy and positive view of sexuality on the part of adults who work with them.

That does not mean that the youth in this category feel that they are receiving all the information about sexuality which they need from their congregational experiences. These youth, like others who participated in the study, did not feel that they received the total range of information or guidance from the congregation which they needed in relation to sexuality, dating, marriage, and parenting. We'll share more about this later in the book.

For youth sharing the characteristics identified above, the percentage who've had sexual intercourse follows:

	9th-10th Grades	11th-12th Grades
Male	6.3%	16.5%
Female	6.7%	15.8%

For youth NOT sharing all the characteristics identified above, the percentage who've had sexual intercourse:

	9th-10th Grades	11th-12th Grades
Male	14.4%	33.9%
Female	16.7%	31.6%

For all youth participating in the study (combining both the groups identified above), the percentage who've had sexual intercourse:

	9th-10th Grades	11th-12th Grades
Male	12.7%	30.9%
Female	14.7%	28.0%

The 2001 figures from the Youth Risk Behavior Surveillance System (YRBSS) of the National Centers for Disease Control and Prevention indicate a much higher percentage of students who have had sexual intercourse. Overall, 42.9% of teenage females and 48.5% of teenage males in the United States have had sexual intercourse according to the YRBSS figures. Those figures show that 34.4% of 9th graders and 60.5% of 12th graders have had intercourse.

While the percentages of all the youth in our study who have had intercourse are lower than in secular surveys, it is important to note that the sample size of 11th and 12th grade youth was not as large as the sample of 9th and 10th grade youth. It is possible that youth who drop out of congregational activity in the later years of high school may be more likely to have had sexual intercourse than those who stay. Many of the youth who are not having intercourse are nevertheless involved in other forms of sexual activity, which we'll share as the chapter progresses.

Here are some of the comments from teens about sexual intercourse:

The first time was horrible. I wondered why anyone would want to do it. My boyfriend. . .just caused me pain. I'll give him credit. When he figured out that it hadn't been good for me, he felt really bad. Then he started working harder so it would be better for me. Now it feels good most of the time, and I like being that close. But I still don't think I've had an orgasm. . . . I don't understand some of my friends who have had sex with four or five different guys. Letting someone inside of you is such an intimate thing. I wouldn't want to do it with someone I didn't love. I do think sex is a gift from God, but I don't see waiting until marriage. Female–Roman Catholic Church

Guilt stops me. We probably shouldn't do everything that we do, but I draw the line at intercourse. You can't undo that. I don't know if I'll wait until marriage or not, but I'm not going to do it in high school. Female–Unitarian Universalist Church

Everyone makes too big a thing out of sex. It's fun. It's a way to be close. It doesn't require a lifetime commitment. The first couple of girls I did it with, did the whole enchilada, I made a mistake in not being clear. Now I let the girl know that this isn't a marriage proposal. It's sex. If she doesn't want to do it, that's fine. But don't be expecting an engagement ring. Male–Independent Christian Church

I don't think I've had an orgasm. The earth never shakes. I don't quiver and moan like my boyfriend does. Sometimes I wonder why I keep doing it. Am I afraid of losing him? Is it a habit now that I can't break? It doesn't do that much for me, and I get filled with guilt. Female–Independent Baptist

My sister is two years older than me. We agreed that we weren't going to have sex until we got married. We aren't the same on what we think it's okay to do though. My sister admits that she and her guy do about anything except intercourse. I don't want to do that. I get aroused just from a kiss and a hug or from dancing. If I let him touch my breasts, I'm afraid my control will slide away. Female–American Baptist Church

*I don't know how to describe it, but it's wonderful. I feel
wide awake and exhausted all at once. More awake than
awake. More tired than tired. I don't see how there can
be anything wrong with this. God made us this way.*
Female–United Methodist Church

*Muslims have this thing of saving themselves for marriage.
That is, the girls are supposed to. It's a different story for
boys. So we get the boys pressuring us for the sex that
adults tell us we shouldn't give. Then the boys will end
up going with outsiders so they can have sex but still want
to come back to a nice Muslim girl to get married. My girl
friends and I feel resentful of the double standard, but
most of us go along with it.* Female–Muslim

*I'm not ready for intercourse. We've found a lot of ways
to give pleasure to each other that don't involve the risk
of pregnancy or disease. We like to dry hump. We get
all the way to orgasm but keep our clothes on. Is that
wrong?* Male–Missouri Synod Lutheran Church

*I have so many friends who have messed up their lives
by getting pregnant. Our youth pastor reminds us that
there may be safer sex but there's no such thing as SAFE
sex. I'll do a lot of things, but nobody is going to stick his
dick in me before a wedding ceremony. Forget it. Jesus
doesn't want it, and I don't want it.* Female–African
Methodist Episcopal Church

Oral Sex

The extent of sexual activity by the youth in our study is
greater than reflected by the statistics for intercourse only. Our
study shows that youth who are active in faith-based
institutions, while less likely than the general youth population
to have had intercourse, are nevertheless participating in other
sexual behaviors. As we have shared the study results in some
settings, many clergy and other congregational leaders have been
particularly surprised by the numbers of youth who are having
oral sex.

The Thursday, November 16, 2000 issue of *USA Today* has an
article about anecdotal evidence that oral sex may be on the

increase among young people and that many of them don't see it as "having sex." A recent report from the Alan Guttmacher Institute also deals with this issue. Oprah Winfrey's show on May 7, 2002 had teens and parents talking about oral sex, which the youth saw as being increasingly common.

Little research information has been published on teens and oral sex. When we were designing our own study, we were surprised by how few secular studies of teens had included questions on this topic. Our own data is some of the first to be released. Oral sex is discussed in the National Survey of Adolescents and Young Adults: Sexual Health Knowledge, Attitudes, and Experience, which was published by the Kaiser Family Foundation. That study indicates that one-third of adolescents have had oral sex.

The figures for oral sex in our study are for that activity with a member of the opposite sex. Oral sex in the context of a homosexual relationship was not covered in the survey. The number of items related to explicit homosexual behavior had to be limited in order to gain the cooperation of clergy in some of the more fundamentalist congregations. The youth who are having oral sex are not always the same ones who have had intercourse. Some have had intercourse but not oral sex; some have had oral sex but not intercourse; and some have had both oral sex and intercourse:

Intercourse and Oral Sex

	Intercourse	Oral Sex	Intercourse and/or Oral Sex
9th-10th Males	12.7%	11.4%	17.3%
9th-10th Females	14.7%	13.6%	19.5%
11th-12th Males	30.9%	28.9%	38.7%
11th-12th Females	29.0%	26.4%	37.6%

In most instances, those who have given oral sex have also received oral sex. Males are slightly more likely than females to have received but not given oral sex. Females are somewhat more likely to have given oral sex but not to have received it. As you can see from the table above, combining those who have given or received oral sex with those who have had intercourse results in a considerably higher level of sexual activity than the figures for intercourse alone. The chart which follows shows the figures in graphic form.

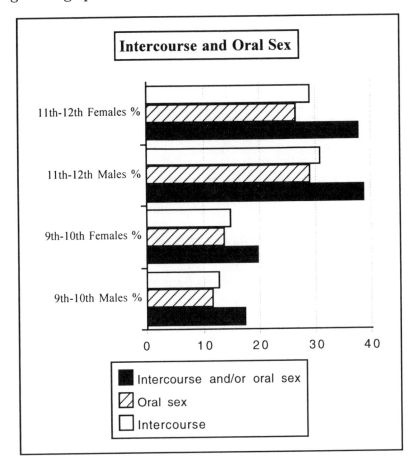

Many of the teens in this study see oral sex as involving not only no danger of pregnancy but also little or no danger of HIV/AIDS or other sexually transmitted diseases. They also make a distinction between intercourse and oral sex in terms of what they see the Scriptures and the congregation teaching.

While they see premarital intercourse being prohibited by the teachings of their tradition, many of the teens feel that the Scriptures and tradition are silent on the matter of oral sex. Here are some of the comments which teens made about oral sex:

We keep trying to do 69. It's hard. How can you focus on your partner when she's doing that to you? We think this is a safe thing to do. No chance of pregnancy and almost no chance of a disease. And the Bible says absolutely nothing about it. I don't think it's wrong. Male–Evangelical Covenant Church

I like it when he does oral sex on me first. Then I'm wet and hot, and it's easier to take him inside me. We just did oral sex until I was able to get the pill. Now we do both. Female–Roman Catholic Church

I was at this party where they played modified spin-the-bottle. When you were "it," you gave oral sex to the first person of the opposite sex the bottle landed on. Then that person would give it a spin and give it to the next person of the opposite sex it landed on. I thought it was gross, but I did it because I wanted to be part of the group. Now I wonder if it was a sin. My friends don't think so, but I'm not sure. Female–Southern Baptist Church

I love it when my girlfriend gives me head. It feels sooooo good. And I feel so close to her when she does it. I would like to do the same for her, but she doesn't want it. She'll dry hump, but she doesn't want to take her clothes off. Male–Church of God

I guess I like oral sex. I mean, I like it fine at the time. It's exciting to give it to him, and it does way more for me than regular sex. But sometimes after we've done it, I feel humiliated or embarrassed by what we've done. Especially when I've been on my knees to do it for him. It's like I've degraded myself. It doesn't feel that way at the time, but it can afterwards. Female–Reformed Church in America

I liked oral sex the first time my girlfriend gave it to me. Then I saw how she felt used and dominated. I won't

*ever push anyone else to do it. Her feeling awful made
me feel awful.* Male–Church of the Brethren

Are Premarital Intercourse and Oral Sex "Wrong"?

We asked youth to respond to some items concerning what
they feel their faith community believes and what their
Scriptures teach concerning intercourse and oral sex. The
following are the statements and the percentage of youth in the
study in agreement with each one:

Are Premarital Intercourse and Oral Sex "Wrong"?

92.8%   My faith community believes that premarital
        intercourse is wrong.

67.3%   The Scriptures of my faith teach that premarital
        intercourse is wrong.

54.1%   I personally believe that premarital intercourse
        is wrong.

65.4%   My faith community believes that oral sex before
        marriage is wrong.

34.7%   My faith community believes that oral sex is wrong
        even for people who are married.

18.9%   The Scriptures of my faith teach that oral sex before
        marriage is wrong.

28.7%   I personally believe that oral sex before marriage is
        wrong.

The teens in this study clearly see a significant difference
between sexual intercourse and oral sex from the standpoint of
the faith community, the Scriptures, and their own beliefs. The
vast majority of the teens in the study believe that their faith
community sees premarital intercourse as wrong, but the
percentage who feel the Scriptures of their faith are clear on the
issue is somewhat lower. Then the percentage who personally

feel premarital intercourse is wrong drops to only a little more than half the respondents. That figure needs to be balanced by the fact that 92.5% indicated agreement with this statement: "Sexual intercourse should only happen between people who have a commitment to each other." Many of the teens are not ready to say that sexual intercourse is only all right in marriage, but there is nothing casual about the view of most of these teens toward intercourse.

Fifty-four percent of the teens personally believe that premarital intercourse is wrong. Only 7% of those who felt personally that it was wrong have had it. The personal conviction that intercourse before marriage is wrong appears to have a greater influence on behavior than simply perceiving that the faith community believes it is wrong.

Oral sex is another matter. The percentage who think that their faith community believes oral sex before marriage is wrong is considerably lower than the number who have that perception concerning their faith community's view of intercourse. Less than one in five of the teens in this study think that the Scriptures of their faith clearly prohibit oral sex before marriage. A large percentage of these congregationally active teens, 71.3%, are not convinced that oral sex before marriage is wrong.

Slightly over a third of the teens, 34.7%, think that their faith community views oral sex as wrong even for persons who are married. Those who belonged to religious traditions that might be described as fundamentalist or conservative were more likely than the other teens in the study to think that their faith community saw oral sex as wrong even in marriage. The teens themselves from those fundamentalist and conservative religious traditions, however, were not more likely to be personally convinced that oral sex is wrong.

Fifty-five percent of the teens agreed with this statement: "A person cannot get a sexually transmitted disease from unprotected oral sex." Thus we have many teens in this study who are not convinced there is anything wrong with having oral sex before marriage and who do not recognize that it is possible to get sexually transmitted diseases from that activity. That's alarming since unprotected oral sex can so readily result in sexually transmitted diseases.

Here are some of the comments of the teens concerning how they feel about premarital intercourse and oral sex from the perspective of faith community and scriptural teachings:

Our youth pastor keeps telling us that it's wrong to have premarital intercourse. But when you read the Scriptures, it isn't all that clear. People got married when they were fourteen and fifteen years old in Bible times, so premarital sex wasn't a concern. Male–Missouri Synod Lutheran

My Sunday school teacher has had a lot of influence on me. She helped me understand how sex is part of God's plan and belongs only in marriage. I'm waiting and happy to be. Female–Nazarene Church

We had a big True Love Waits campaign in my church and my school, but nobody mentioned oral sex until I asked about it. Then I got told that of course it was wrong but not why it was wrong. It won't make you pregnant, and you won't get AIDS. Why is it wrong? The Bible says nothing about it. Female–American Baptist Church

I don't plan to get married until after law school. I just know that I won't be able to go that long without having sex. But I know I'm too young right now. I've only been driving a car for six months. And I wouldn't do it unless I loved the person. Male–African Methodist Episcopal Church

It's clear to me that the church and my parents and my school think sex before marriage is wrong. But no one is all that clear about why it's wrong. I respect these people, but this is a topic we are never able to talk about. Female–United Methodist Church

I go to a Catholic high school. We get lectures from a nun and a priest about this. Well, of course, they don't think we should do anything before getting married. They've made this promise to God to never have sex, so waiting for marriage doesn't seem like a big deal to them. But I love Brian, and we should be able to express our love for each other. The desire is just so strong. *The priest and the nun aren't sitting in the car with us.* Female–Roman Catholic Church

No one wants us to have any information about this. All we get told is the big NO. I'd like to talk more about this. Why shouldn't I have sex before marriage? Where do you draw the lines between kissing and touching and oral sex and intercourse? This is such an important part of life, and we do not get help from adults. Male–Reformed Church

When I think about the responsibility to God and to the person I love, I know that intercourse is a big step. My pastor is right–it belongs in marriage. Male–United Methodist Church

I have the opinion that the faith should have a lot to say about my relationship with a guy. It's not just whether or not to have sex. What about honesty? What about communication? What about touching? What about respecting and being respected? No one helps you with this. The Torah has all these confusing teachings. Which parts really apply to life today? Female–Synagogue (Reformed)

My priest rocks and is not negative on sex. He helped me see how God intends marriage to be. I feel good about myself, and I know I'm worth waiting for. Female–Roman Catholic Church

I had sex with this guy because I thought we were in love. I thought we were going to get married when we were both out of college. It felt right to do it. Then I found out that he was doing it with another girl all the time he was doing it with me. I am such a loser. I've lost something that I can never get back. Female–Missouri Synod Lutheran Church

My pastor and my youth group advisor have taught me to pray about the things that I do–before I do them. When I pray about whether or not to have sex with Tracy, I never get a clear signal that it's all right. Does that mean she's not the person I'll marry? Does that mean it would be a sin to have sex with her even

*if we were going to get married later? I don't know
the answers to the questions, but I do know that it
would be wrong to have sex before I get some kind
of all clear from God.* Male–Christian Church (Disciples
of Christ)

We'll talk more in Chapter Seven about what congregations
are actually doing to help young people relate their faith to their
sexuality, but a few observations are appropriate at this point in
the book:

- Teenagers do care about what they perceive
  their faith communities believe and what the
  Scriptures teach, but teens do not always agree
  with those teachings. And they often do not
  receive the information they need and want
  from their faith communities.

- Most of these teenagers view their faith communities
  and the Scriptures as being fairly silent on the topic
  of oral sex. While the majority of these congregationally active teens have not yet had oral sex, they
  are not convinced that it is "wrong."

- While these religious teens are not all convinced
  that premarital intercourse is a sin, most of them
  are convinced that it only should happen between
  persons who have a commitment to each other.
  They do not see it as a casual activity.

- Many of these teens have not received accurate
  information about the health dangers from oral
  sex. As future chapters will share, they have also
  not received the information they need concerning
  contraception and other aspects of sexual relationships.

- Teenagers who are active in their faith communities
  have received an abstinence message on premarital
  intercourse, but they would like to better understand
  the reasons for the prohibition. They would also like
  to receive considerably more information and guidance
  from their faith communities than they do at the

47

present time about how to relate their sexuality to their spirituality and their relationships with others.

Kissing, Petting, Being Naked

The fact that the majority of these teens are not having premarital intercourse or oral sex does not mean that they are uninvolved in sexual contact. Note the percentages who have been involved in petting (fondling the partner's breasts or genitals) and who have been completely nude with a member of the opposite sex (within the last two years, so that bathtub play as young children is not counted):

Petting
(Fondling a partner's breasts and/or genitals)

Males 9th-10th	Females 9th-10th	Males 11th-12th	Females 11th-12th
28.8%	30.7%	71.6%	70.9%

Being completely nude with a member of the opposite sex

Males 9th-10th	Females 9th-10th	Males 11th-12th	Females 11th-12th
16.3%	17.6%	50.3%	47.2%

The percentage who have been involved in petting and who have been nude with a member of the opposite sex are much higher for 11th and 12th graders than for 9th and 10th graders. As teens go out more and have more opportunities for privacy, these behaviors increase.

Those statistics raise some obvious questions. Did we ask them to distinguish between fondling the breasts and fondling the genitals? No. We should have. Have those who have been completely nude with a member of the opposite sex all been involved in making out or petting? Yes, with the exception of six persons. Have all those who have had intercourse or oral sex been completely nude with a member of the opposite sex? No. A few who have had intercourse and more who have had oral sex have done so without taking off all their clothes.

The written comments on the surveys, the interviews with selected teens, and the discussion of the survey results with some teens have pointed to another area of sexual activity which we didn't directly cover with a survey question and should have: what teenagers call "dry humping." This happens when teens have direct genital-to-genital contact without skin-to-skin contact in the process. They keep their clothes on and rub against each other, generally to the point of ejaculation for the boy. Because there is no exchange of fluids, the teens see this as a way to avoid the risk of pregnancy or disease. Some of them also see it as an activity not clearly prohibited by Scripture or by faith community teaching.

There are variations on dry humping. Some do it wearing street clothes. Some do it on or near the beach wearing swimming suits. Some strip to their underwear. In some instances, the male will remove his underwear, but the female leaves her underwear on. There are some parts of the country where the phrase dry humping is used to describe the intimate contact in certain styles of dancing; but that contact, while highly arousing, does not usually lead to orgasm on the dance floor.

Some media stories have focused on the growing popularity of coed sleepovers (as opposed to the more traditional same-sex slumber party). Our study did not include any objective questions about coed sleepovers, but we did have over two hundred youth who offered comments about coed sleepovers. About three-fourths of those commenting expressed resentment of adult suspicion of coed sleepovers and maintained that kids did not have sex at the sleepovers in which they participated. Nine percent of those commenting on the topic said they knew of people having sex at coed sleepovers. Youth, pastors, and adult youth advisors were quick to point out in focus groups that males and females always sleep in separate areas at congregationally sponsored lock-ins. Lock-ins are overnight retreats held in the church or synagogue at which youth rest for part of the night in sleeping bags or simply stay up all night participating in a variety of discussions and activities.

And what about kissing? Yes, there's certainly plenty of that going on. Some teens, however, kiss their friends of the opposite

49

sex on the cheek even if not involved in any kind of dating or going out relationship. Thus it's important to be cautious in interpreting what teens say about kissing. Almost all the teens in the study have kissed a member of the opposite sex, but that doesn't always mean the same thing. The percentage of teens who have been involved in kissing that included the insertion of the tongue into the mouth of the other person ran about the same as for petting (around 30% for 9th and 10th graders and 70% for 11th and 12th graders).

We asked the youth in the study if they thought it was all right to kiss on a first or second date. Among 9th and 10th grade males, 96.2% said that it was; 93.8% of the female in those years of school said that it was. Among 11th and 12th grade males, 97.4% said that it was; 94.1% of the females that age said it was. Some females, however, offered the observation that males who did not make a move for a kiss on a first or second date made a very positive impression. They felt more respected by males who were not in a hurry to initiate that kind of contact.

Here are a few of the comments the youth offered concerning petting, being nude with the opposite sex, and related experiences:

I like my neck being kissed. . . and his nibbling on my ear. Doing that and holding each other close feels so good. That's enough for me. I don't need more. Female–United Church of Christ

Feeling up is the big thing with my boyfriend. He's a real breast man. If he did it more gently, I'd like it. But it does more for him than for me. Female–Roman Catholic Church

We like to get naked and touch each other and be close. We've started rubbing each other all the way to the big O, and I love that. I don't see a need for us to do anything more. Male–United Methodist Church

Dry humping is a big thing in our school. You don't get pregnant. You don't get a disease. You get to be close and give pleasure. . . . Once you've done it a few times, I think you start to want more. I'd like to feel

her skin next to mine. But I respect her and won't push it. Male–Roman Catholic Church

The youth also had some interesting comments to share related to arousal, which can of course come in a multitude of ways:

When I watch some movies, like American Pie, which I've seen like 20 times, I get horny. I really want to do something by myself or with someone else. Female– Synagogue (Reformed)

I wonder if I could be oversexed or something. I go through the day getting turned on by so many different things. By good looking girls, by good looking teachers, by things I read, by movies. I have this English teacher who is so hot. She's maybe 25 years old and looks like Cameron Diaz. I'm not kidding. One day she walked by my desk and put a hand on my shoulder for just a second. I got such a boner I didn't know if I would be able to leave when the bell rang. Male–Pentecostal Holiness Church

My youth pastor gave me some great advice. He said you'd be big as a house if you ate each time you felt hungry and that you'd be exhausted if you had sex each time you felt aroused. The arousal is normal, but it doesn't mean you have to do something. Male–Presbyterian Church USA

I thought I was abnormal until we had this good discussion in Sunday school. You can get aroused by all kinds of things. I knew that was true for me, but I never heard anyone talk about it. I had read this article about girls not getting aroused by as many things or as fast as guys. But from what our Sunday school teacher and some others in the class said, that isn't always true. I felt so much better after the class. I was about to write that I needed that more than Bible study, but we got into it talking about David and Bathsheba. Female–Evangelical Lutheran Church

Masturbation

Some religious traditions teach that masturbation is wrong. The majority of the teens in our study, however, have masturbated. There are no significant differences in the frequency of masturbation among the major religious traditions with the exception of Muslim teens. Female Muslims were less likely than females in other traditions to practice masturbation. Male Muslims did not show different rates of masturbation than other teens in the study.

Percentage Who Masturbate

Males 9th-10th	Females 9th-10th	Males 11th-12th	Females 11th-12th
81.2%	60.8%	89.4%	71.3%%

Here are comments from some teens about masturbation:

Sometimes I worry about being addicted to masturbation. I do it almost every night. I don't have a girlfriend, and I know it would be wrong to have sex with her if I did have one. What I do for myself keeps me from being too frustrated, but I don't talk to anyone about doing it. You can talk with guys in my school about intercourse or oral sex or whatever, but no one owns up to what they do under the covers at night. Male–United Church of Christ

[Masturbation] is how I get pleasure, and it makes it easier not to go too far with a boy. I'll touch tongue with a guy I like but nothing more than that. No touching the breasts, and no taking clothes off. Female–Roman Catholic Church

When I play with myself, I'm thinking of Buffy the Vampire Killer. She's so hot. There are reruns at 11 pm week nights, and I like to watch the show right before going to bed. Male–Progressive Baptist Church

I've found some creative uses for the shower nozzle. It feels so good, no one knows what I'm doing, and then I just finish cleaning myself. I thought I would stop when Bobby and I started having sex, but it still feels good. We don't get to have sex all that often. Female–Mennonite Church

*My church teaches that masturbation is wrong. But
everything that I've read says that it's a normal thing
that almost everybody does. There's nothing in the
Bible that convinces me there's something wrong with
giving yourself pleasure. Isn't it a lot better to do it
with yourself than to have premarital intercourse?*
Male–Missouri Synod Lutheran Church

Reflections

Prior to the publication of this book, the data has been shared only in limited settings. What we have generally found is that adults who are familiar with the data from secular studies on teens are surprised that the level of premarital intercourse among teens in this study is so low. Clergy and adult youth advisors in congregations, however, are surprised both by the level of premarital intercourse and even more by the levels of oral sex, petting, and being nude with the opposite sex. These teens definitely are sexually active.

As the book progresses, we'll talk more about the ways in which teens wish they received more guidance from their faith communities concerning dating and sexuality. Most of them accurately perceive that their faith communities believe premarital intercourse is wrong, but they would appreciate considerably more help than just the prohibition. Because the teens themselves would like that help, there are opportunities for most of our congregations to do considerably more than they are at present.

Sexuality and Spirituality
Guidelines for Religious People

We visited with youth in five different congregational settings about guidelines for decision-making by people who want to relate their sexuality to their spirituality. Would you make any changes in the list?

1. A religious person recognizes that there is no such thing as a "just physical" relationship. Persons cannot be treated as objects. You must be concerned about the mental, emotional, and spiritual dimensions of those to whom you relate.
2. A religious person recognizes that sexual intercourse is most proper and fulfilling within the context of marriage.
3. A religious person will not use dishonesty, threats, or manipulation to gain his or her sexual desires with another person.
4. A religious person recognizes that sexual intimacy should not develop more quickly than intimacy in communication and in shared experiences.
5. A religious person who chooses to engage in sexual intercourse will take appropriate steps to avoid an unwanted pregnancy and sexually transmitted diseases.
6. A religious person recognizes that heavy petting and oral sex represent an extremely high level of physical intimacy and that oral sex carries the risk of sexually transmitted diseases.
7. A religious person recognizes that sex is a gift from God and should be enjoyed.
8. A religious person does not gossip about the real or the assumed sexual experiences of other persons and recognizes that such gossip can hurt people deeply.
9. A religious person is not afraid to talk about sexual concerns and recognizes that clear communication is essential to a good sexual relationship.
10. A religious person respects the right of others to hold and express differing values on sexual issues.
11. A religious person prays for guidance in sexual decision-making.
12. A religious person is at least as concerned about his or her partner's pleasure as about personal enjoyment.

Chapter Three
Abstinence

[N]o longer on the defensive and apologizing for their choices, virgins are expressing a new pride and are starting to stand up for themselves and be counted. Like the women who say yes, those who say no are operating from a basic ethic of the sexual revolution: the right to control their own sexuality.

Paula Kamen
Her Way

Abstinence

Our hope is that the sexual ethics of teenagers will grow out of Scripture and the teachings of their congregations and parents–rather than out of the sexual revolution as suggested in the above quote from Paula Kamen's intriguing book about young adult women. Kamen's view is that young women who are choosing to be virgins are doing so without apology. The teenagers in our study are younger than those to whom Kamen is referring, but the majority of them have not yet had sexual intercourse. While some of them have not yet had the opportunity for premarital intercourse, many have intentionally decided that they do not wish to engage in it at the present time. Here are some comments from teens about abstaining from intercourse and choosing virginity:

I want to be a virgin when I'm married. I want that first night together to be the most beautiful in my life.
Female–Church of God

If you have sex with every person you go out with, then what's left to share with the one person you decide to marry? Male–American Baptist Church

My youth advisor told me that she'd had sex before she was married and was sorry that she had. She didn't think it made her an awful person, but she would have liked herself better if she'd waited. I don't want to

make the same mistake. Female–Evangelical Lutheran Church

The body is the temple of God. The Bible's clear on this. That means that you want to use your body in a way that is pleasing to God. Waiting until marriage for sex is part of honoring God through the body. Male–United Methodist Church

I plan to wait on marriage until I've finished college and have a career started. I don't know if I'll wait until then to have intercourse, but I do know I'm not ready now. And I resent it when a guy thinks he has it coming because he pays for a movie and pizza. Female–Roman Catholic Church

If Mary was a virgin when Jesus was conceived, wasn't Joseph too? Our youth pastor says that virginity is for males and females. I wouldn't want to marry a person who had intercourse with other people, and I need to meet my own standard. Male–Presbyterian Church U.S.A.

Virginity is a choice. You don't owe anyone an explanation. I choose it to honor God, my parents, and myself. I don't think it makes me better than people who make a different choice, but I also don't think it makes me weird. Female–Synagogue [Reformed]

In our study, 41.7% of the ninth grade females and 32.3% of the ninth grade males indicated that they are committed to waiting until they are married before having sexual intercourse. That percentage of agreement declines with each year in school. Among twelfth graders, 22.8% of the females and 17.6% of the males are committed to waiting until they are married before having sexual intercourse. That means 77% of these young women and 82% of these young men are considering the possibility that they will have sex before marriage.

The fact that the majority of the teens are not committing themselves to waiting until marriage before having intercourse does not mean that they take this activity lightly. As shared in the last chapter, 92.5% of the teens in our study indicated agreement with this statement: "Sexual intercourse should only happen between people who have a commitment to each other."

Many of the teens did not say that sexual intercourse only belongs in marriage, but there is nothing casual about the view of most of these teens toward intercourse.

Abstinence and Comprehensive Sexuality Education

How do the leaders of faith-based institutions view the role of congregations in encouraging abstinence from sexual inter-course until marriage? We asked the clergy and adult youth leaders who participated in our study to indicate how they felt about teaching both abstinence and comprehensive sexuality education.

It's important to point out that most professional sexuality educators see comprehensive sexuality education including the teaching of abstinence. We discovered in the focus groups that we conducted before doing the survey that clergy and other adult youth teachers and advisors generally did not see comprehensive sexuality education including abstinence. For the purposes of our survey of clergy and other adult leaders, we described comprehensive sexuality education as including factual knowledge about the body and sexuality, scriptural and theological background, relationship issues, pregnancy and sexually transmitted disease prevention, and guidance in decision-making. Here's how the clergy and other adult leaders responded:

4.2%   Agreed that faith-based institutions should teach comprehensive sexuality education to teenagers and did not check teaching abstinence

30.3%   Agreed that faith-based institutions should teach teenagers to abstain from sexual intercourse and did not check teaching comprehensive sexuality education

61.5%   Agreed that faith-based institutions should teach both comprehensive sexuality education and abstinence

4.0%   Agreed that all sexuality education should be in the home and not in the faith-based institution

In Chapter Seven, we'll share in detail what clergy and adult youth leaders think about the form that sexuality education of teenagers should take. At this point, we want to point out that 91.8% of the clergy and other adults participating in the study think that it's important to teach abstinence. The minority who did not agree that it was important to teach abstinence either felt that only comprehensive sexuality education should be taught or that no sexuality education of teens should happen in faith-based institutions.

A substantial percentage, 61.5%, felt that both abstinence and comprehensive sexuality education should be taught by faith-based institutions. This result generated some heated debate in a couple of group settings where these results were shared. Here are some of the comments from clergy and other adult leaders about the teaching of both abstinence and comprehensive sexuality education:

- *If you teach them abstinence and then teach them about sexuality and birth control, you've sent a mixed message. It's like saying, "You really shouldn't do it. But if you are going to do it, then you should know about birth control."*

- *We don't do a good job of teaching abstinence or teaching something more comprehensive. Anything we would do would be an improvement.*

- *The culture has these kids horribly confused. The church needs to say a clear, loud "No" to sexual intercourse before marriage. If you teach them anything else, you are confusing the issue.*

- *We did the True Love Waits program in several congregations and a couple of schools. It seemed to have impact, but it's hard to know long term. The weakness of the program, I thought, was that the youth aren't taught enough about their sexuality to help them know how to handle the drives that are natural in everyone. Abstinence is good, but we need to give them more information than just that.*

- *I think synagogues and churches have a responsibility not just to help teens with their decision-making today but also to help them be prepared for the decisions about sex*

*they'll be making as adults. Almost all of them are going
to get married. They're going to be in sexual relationships.
We should help them prepare for that. Teaching them to
abstain while they are in high school is fine, but they aren't
going to be in high school forever.*

- *I'll tell you what doing abstinence and comprehensive
education is like. It's just like telling them it's wrong to
shoot a gun and then giving them classes in how to handle
firearms.*

- *You can go through your whole life without ever needing
to handle a gun. You can't live one day of your life without
being a sexual person. We have a responsibility to help
teens have the information they need.*

- *If abstinence is going to work, then it has to be put in a
positive kind of way. You have to be saving yourself
for something rather than just giving up what you think
will give you pleasure right now.*

- *I'm convinced that you can do the best job of teaching
teens to abstain when you give them the full information
about being a sexual person and a child of God.*

- *If we care about them, then we have to teach them both.
I am very concerned about where our teens are learning
about sex. They're learning from their friends and from
the media–not exactly great sources of accurate   information. I support sexuality education in the schools, but we're
fooling ourselves in the religious community if we think
that does the job. They need a moral and ethical frame-
work for sexual decisions. That has to come from the
religious community and from parents.*

- *The teen years are a time of preparation for life. We give
them at least some of the tools they need to buy a home
and run a business, but they aren't going to do that for
several years. We need to give them the tools for living
as sexual persons, even though we hope they'll wait until
they are married or at least older before having intercourse.*

- *Why do we teach abstinence in our church rather than
something comprehensive? Because everyone supports*

> *teaching abstinence, but people aren't sure how much more to offer.*

Pledges

Given the very large percentage of leaders who favor teaching abstinence (on its own or as a part of comprehensive sexuality education), it's not surprising that this is the approach which is most comfortable for many congregations. A movement called True Love Waits has been especially popular. That movement seeks to have teens sign this pledge:

> *Believing that true love waits, I make a commitment to God, myself, my family and my friends, my future mate and my future children to be sexually abstinent from this day until the day I enter a biblical marriage relationship.*

True Love Waits originated in the Southern Baptist denomination but has become a movement which is not exclusive to any denomination. About 90 organizations participate in this ministry, including denominations and crisis pregnancy centers, as well as some popular Christian recording artists. In our survey, we found that youth in many different Christian denominations have participated in this movement, including Roman Catholic, United Methodist, Southern Baptist, Disciples of Christ, Episcopal, Missouri Synod Lutheran, Evangelical Lutheran, and Pentecostal teens. While congregations cooperate and are generally the driving force behind the movement in a particular geographical area, the program itself sometimes comes to life through the school system and will reach teens who are not connected with any faith-based institution as well as those who are active in congregations.

From the time of the initial planning process for our study, we were very interested in what relationship we would discover between pledges like the one teens make in the True Love Waits movement and their sexual activity. We had hoped for a stronger connection between the making of such a pledge and abstinence from sexual intercourse than we actually found.

Although 19% of the youth responding to the survey have taken a pledge to remain a virgin until marriage, that subgroup was not any more or less likely than others in our sample to have had sexual intercourse or to have experienced or caused pregnancy. The promotion of abstinence by the faith-based institution does have an impact, when combined with other characteristics as noted earlier in this book. On the basis of our study, the taking of a pledge itself does not have impact greater than the promotion of abstinence in the congregation.

That finding seems in conflict with a report by Peter Bearman and Hannah Brückner based on an analysis of teenagers in the National Longitudinal Study of Adolescent Health. Their report, published in the *American Journal of Sociology*, indicates that teens who made virginity pledges delayed sex about eighteen months longer than others. There seem to us at least three reasons for the apparent difference.

First, our study looked at formal virginity or abstinence pledges as one of several religious variables. Most youth in our sample were highly religious, so the relative impact of the pledge might be expected to be different than in the more secular sample of the National Longitudinal Study.

Second, the overall frequency of sexual intercourse among the teenagers in our study was much lower than most other studies have reported. The impact of a pledge might well be different on these youth.

Third, the impact of the pledge, as reported by Bearman and Brückner, is greatest when it is not too popular in the school–when forty or fifty percent of a school takes the pledge, it no longer has impact. We can't speak to the school situation from our data; but most of the youth in our sample who took such a pledge were in a congregation in which most of the other teens did so–in fact there was tremendous peer pressure for them to take that step.

Some teens who have made virginity pledges have nevertheless had intercourse and even become pregnant or impregnated someone. Here are a few comments from teens in our study who are in that situation:

At times I have a lot of guilt because I made the pledge and then broke it. I didn't know how hard it was going to be to keep the pledge. I don't so much feel bad about

*having sex as I do about breaking my word. I would
be sick if my parents and pastor knew what I've done.*
Female–Southern Baptist Church

*I felt like we were forced into making the pledge. All
these cards got put up on the bulletin board in the church.
Our church isn't that big. If your card didn't go up there,
people were going to know. You had to make the pledge
or catch s - - - from the pastor and your parents. Most
of us knew it didn't mean anything.* Male–Missouri
Synod Lutheran Church

*I broke the pledge, but I'm still glad I made it. It kept
me from having sex too early. Before my boyfriend and
I had sex, I thought about it and prayed. I feel like God
released me from my promise. My boyfriend and I are
in love, and we're going to get married. Having sex with
him isn't the same as it would have been with anyone else.*
Female–Disciples of Christ

*I broke the pledge, and I'm sorry I did. I thought the two
of us were in love and were going to get married. Turns
out he was having sex with another person the nights we
weren't together. I thought he was doing homework. . . .
True Love Waits talks about being able to have a second
chance. You can pray to God and like become a virgin
again. That's what I'm trying to do.* Female–Church of
God

*The pledge thing didn't work for me. I remembered it for
maybe a couple of months. Then things with my boyfriend
just kept going further and further. We had sex. I got
pregnant. I had an abortion. So much for the pledge. . . .
The pledge is only going to work if you are already a
good person. For someone like me, the pledge won't
make a difference.* Female–Evangelical Covenant Church

In sharing the previous comments, we aren't trying to discourage congregations and communities from involvement in programs like True Love Waits. We do, however, want to share a couple of suggestions for those who work with such programs:

- Consideration should be given to providing more comprehensive sexuality education along with the promotion of abstinence and virginity pledges. The young people who made the pledges and still had sex certainly would have benefited from more information about topics like contraception and sexually transmitted disease prevention.

- Congregations which encourage virginity pledges need to be aware of the fact that not all who make the pledges will end up keeping them. Discussions with teens need to cover acceptance, forgiveness, and second chances.

As shared in the last chapter, we did identify a subgroup of teens who were significantly less likely to have had sexual intercourse than the other teens in our study. Those teens (1,093 or 18.8%) share these characteristics:

- They attend religious services one or more times a week.
- They pray daily.
- They have involvement in at least one congregational group besides religious education and worship.
- They say that the teachings of the congregation and/or the Scriptures have "a lot of influence" on their sexual decisions.
- They say the congregation has provided information on how to make sexual decisions and on what the Scriptures says about sexuality.
- They feel a strong connection with congregational leaders who work with youth.
- They feel a strong connection with other youth in the congregation.
- They feel the adults who work with them portray sex in a healthy and positive way.
- They say their congregation encourages abstinence from intercourse for high school aged people.

The encouragement of abstinence is a factor, but it is only one factor for this group of youth who were especially unlikely to have had intercourse. All of the factors are positive in nature: strong attendance and involvement, strong connections with other youth and with adults who work with youth, and what they see as a healthy and positive view of sexuality on the part of adults who work with them.

We'll talk more about sexuality education in congregational settings as the book progresses, particularly in Chapter Seven. In closing this chapter, we want to share a cautionary reminder of one of the limitations of our study. There may be significant differences between those faith-based institutions which agreed to take part in our study and those which did not choose to do so. We suspect that the congregations which did participate have a greater openness in talking about sexuality with teens than those which did not. That may have an impact on all of our results–including the relatively low rate of sexual intercourse and the apparent lack of influence of virginity pledges.

More than Abstinence

As we'll share in greater detail in Chapter Seven, there is a tremendous gulf between the number of faith-based institutions in which clergy and adult leaders feel there should be comprehensive sexuality education and the number of congregations in which that education actually takes place. In the 8% of congregations in our study which offered information on contraception, no instances of teen pregnancy were reported. Our study suggests that providing information on contraception did not make teens either more or less likely to have sexual intercourse–but it did make them less likely to become pregnant if they had intercourse.

In a report called *No Easy Answers,* Douglas Kirby shares the results of a careful overview of programs designed to reduce teen pregnancy. Kirby looked at a wide range of programs used in schools, shelters, and detention centers, though none of these are religious programs. Kirby's observations are important for those who are concerned that sexuality education may have a negative influence on teens. He writes: "Evaluations of these programs strongly support the conclusion that sexuality and HIV education curricula do not increase sexual intercourse, either by hastening the onset of intercourse, increasing the frequency of intercourse, or increasing the number of sexual partners" [p. 25].

In almost all the congregations in our study, the teens who responded shared a desire for more sexuality education to be provided. Consider these comments:

*We all know that the church and our parents don't want
us to have sexual intercourse. Not while in high school,
maybe not while in college, and maybe not ever. Just
kidding. It's okay when you get married. But we need
to know more than that. If the answer to intercourse is no,
what about oral sex? What is it okay to do? When is it
okay to do it?* Male–United Church of Christ

*Abstinence. That's the big answer to alcohol, drugs,
and sex. But with sex, we need to know a lot more than
we do. Where do people expect us to learn these things?
Television? The movies?* Female–Roman Catholic Church

*The youth group advisors at my church have tried to provide
us with the facts about sex. But in addition to that, we need
help understanding what the Bible says. Our advisors feel
like totally inadequate to cover that, and no one would want
to listen to our pastor.* Male–Presbyterian Church U.S.A.

*When I was afraid I was pregnant, I went to our pastor
for help. He taught me so many things about the Bible and
about sex. It turned out that I wasn't pregnant, but I sure am
glad I spoke to him. The rest of the high school students need
the same information, but our teachers are scared to do it in
Sunday school.* Female–African Methodist Episcopal Church

*We have a debate right now about how much youth should
be told about sex. Some want to share all the facts with us,
and some think it will get us in trouble. I'm disappointed that
more isn't being done to help us.* Male–Unitarian Universalist

Our conviction, based on the survey results, the focus
groups, and discussion of the results in various settings, is that
a focus on abstinence alone or on virginity pledges does not
constitute an adequate approach to sexuality education in
faith-based institutions. The promotion of abstinence needs to
be a part of comprehensive sexuality education, which in
religious settings should include the relationship of spirituality
to sexuality. The reasons for this conviction:

- Formal virginity pledges in our study did not correlate
  with higher or lower rates of sexual intercourse. We
  don't want to discourage such pledges, since the Peter
  Bearman and Hannah Brückner study suggests that

they may have an impact on less congregationally active teens than those in our study. But we feel that congregations should not rely exclusively on that strategy, especially since, among the teens in our study, the formal pledge had no greater impact than the encouragement of abstinence without a formal pledge.

- The subgroup of teens in our study who showed significantly lower rates of sexual intercourse shared a number of characteristics. The fact that they saw their congregations encouraging abstinence was only one of those characteristics. While not all of the congregations of this subgroup were offering comprehensive sexuality education, they certainly were including some elements of that, including the provision of information on how to make sexual decisions and on what the Scriptures say about sexuality.

- Our study shows that when congregations provide information on contraception to teens, it does not result in teens being either more or less likely to have sexual intercourse–but it does make them less likely to become pregnant.

- Most teens are going to marry. Intercourse and other sexual activities will be part of their lives. Churches and other faith-based institutions should help youth have the necessary information for a lifetime of healthy sexuality.

- The teens themselves want their congregations to do more to help them with sexual decision-making. That was true for teens who have had sexual intercourse and also for teens who have not. Since teens themselves are requesting more comprehensive sexuality education, congregations should respond positively.

Chapter Four
Contraception

*I showed the youth group a video that talked about
all contraception having a failure rate. Later a sixteen-
year-old girl came to me afraid she was pregnant. The
video had made her think there was no point in using
contraception. The purpose of the video was to encourage
abstinence—not to tell teens not to use contraception. . . .
I'm thankful she talked to me. I told her that if she was
going to have intercourse, she had to protect herself
against pregnancy and disease.*

Minister
Southern Baptist Church

Pregnancy and Abortion

The Southern Baptist minister quoted above had been
committed to the promotion of abstinence in the youth group,
and he had intentionally provided opportunities for teens to talk
about sex. The video, produced by a prominent parachurch
organization, had carried a strong abstinence message, telling
teens that there is no such thing as "safe sex." (Parachurch
organizations, for those not familiar with the jargon, exist to
serve congregations but are not officially connected with a
specific denomination. Some are operated for profit, and some
are nonprofit. Christian Community, which developed the
resource you are holding, is a nonprofit parachurch organization.)

The producers of the video hoped, as did the pastor, that
statistics on failure rates for condoms and the pill would instill a
sense of caution in teens. This pastor had not considered the
possibility that in promoting abstinence they might be
discouraging contraception. In this case, the openness of the
pastor to talking with youth about sex, caused the teenager to
confide in him and gain understanding.

While the adult leaders we surveyed in congregations and
visited with in focus groups virtually all feel that high school

students are too young to be having sexual intercourse, the reality is that many teens, including those active in congregations, are choosing to do so. Those teens who do choose to have intercourse need protection against pregnancy and sexually transmitted diseases. Our study found that many teens who are having sexual intercourse are not using contraception and also that many have inaccurate information about protection against pregnancy and sexually transmitted diseases. As those of us who are religious leaders care about youth and their future, these are areas of significant concern.

Among the teens in our study who are having sexual intercourse, 27.4% did not use any form of contraception the first time; and 19.5% did not use contraception the most recent time. Thus it is not surprising that some youth who participate in faith-based institutions have been pregnant or have gotten someone pregnant (percentages of all youth; not just sexually active youth):

	9th-10th Grades	11th-12th Grades
Male	1.6%	3.1%
Female	1.8%	2.8%

When the percentages are looked at in terms of the youth who are having intercourse, they become more alarming with 12.9% of sexually active 9th-10th grade females and 9.9% of sexually active 11th-12th grade females reporting a pregnancy. It is also important to note that some females active in faith-based institutions who become pregnant may drop out of activity in the faith-based institution and thus are not part of our data.

In the National Survey of Adolescents and Young Adults: Sexual Health Knowledge, Attitudes, and Experiences study, 8% of adolescents reported that they or a partner have been pregnant [Kaiser Family Foundation, 2003]. That percentage is considerably higher than we found among these teens who are very involved in their faith-based institutions.

Half of the females responding to the survey who had become pregnant had ended it with an abortion. Several teens who had abortions commented that it was the only acceptable alternative given the views of their families and congregations about unwed mothers. Here's what two teenage females said about dealing with pregnancy:

I could not believe it when I got pregnant. We used a condom each time we did it except once. Apparently once was all it took! My church is pro-life and very, very down on abortion. I've helped people pass out pro-life brochures in front of a Planned Parenthood. But when I got pregnant, after I got over the shock, I didn't see many options. I shouldn't have had sex with the guy, and I sure didn't want to mess up my life by marrying him.

If I'd gone ahead and had the baby, people in my parish would have been so disappointed in me. The shame would just have killed me. And it would have been the same at school–it's a Catholic school.

I finally broke down and talked to my mother. She didn't believe in abortion either, but she agreed with me that it was the only option that made sense. And we never did tell my father that I had been pregnant or had an abortion. He couldn't have handled it. He would probably have kicked me out of the house. . . .

So now I live with this big secret. I think in my heart that God has forgiven me for what I did–for having sex so early and having the abortion. But some of my friends and the people in my parish would never forgive me if they knew. Junior– Roman Catholic Church

My guy and I had the pregnancy coming. As I look back now, I can see that we really asked for it. We didn't use any kind of birth control. Our church is so down on having sex that we were trying not to. But we'd starting making out without clothes, and then we did oral sex which didn't seem like it was quite sex. And then we'd end up doing the "real thing."

My pastor teaches that abortion is murder–one of the worst sins you can commit. My parents feel the same way. But if I had gone ahead and had the baby, there is no way that I could ever have gone to church again. I can't imagine what my parents would do if they knew. I had this older friend who acted like she was my mother so I could get the abortion. Without her I don't know what I would have done. . . . I don't know how God feels about me now. The Bible says that we can be forgiven anything, and I know I've heard our pastor say that. But people would think I was a murderer if they knew. Maybe I am. I just couldn't make myself destroy my whole life by having the child. Sophomore–Free Methodist Church

Here are quotes from three girls who were pregnant and kept their babies:

While I was pregnant, people at church were superficially friendly, but I could tell how much they disapproved. I finally stopped coming until I had the baby. People could deal with the baby more easily than with my being pregnant. Senior–Christian Church, Disciples of Christ

Most people in my church were pretty supportive. The older people were better than people my age. I think the older people disapproved more, but they covered it up well. People my age didn't know what to say. And I think a couple of the girls were afraid I might go after their guys because I'd be wanting a husband. Like that's so totally not where I am at. Junior–United Methodist Church

I went ahead and got married, but it's been a rough journey for us. We've both been able to stay in high school because our parents help us so much, but college is going to be impossible for both of us to do at the same time. . . . He'll have to go to a community college, and I'll have to get a job. We're lucky that our mothers will probably keep providing child care. But we can't ask them to do everything for us financially. We have to start standing on our own. . . . The church has been very supportive to us. People have been wonderful. We haven't felt judged or anything. I'm the one who judges us dumb. Senior–American Baptist Church

African American females responding to the survey were somewhat more likely than white females to become pregnant, but they were less likely than white females to have abortions. Those African American females who were pregnant, for the most part, reported experiencing a high degree of supportiveness from their congregations. Most of the white teenagers who had been pregnant did not feel supported by their congregations. When these results were shared with a group of clergy, one African American minister made this observation:

I can't speak for others, but teenage pregnancy is a big
problem among the black teenagers I know. We in the
church aren't doing enough to help them avoid getting
pregnant, but we have some experience in dealing with
them once they are. . . . Maybe ten or fifteen years ago,
we would have shamed them out of the church. We don't
do that now. We know they need us, and that's what the
church is about.

In two of our focus groups, however, we had African American pastors who talked about teenage girls who were pregnant being pushed out of the church.

There were almost no pregnancies reported among those involved in Jewish or Islamic congregations, and those subgroups also had the lowest rates of sexual intercourse. Jewish youth having sexual intercourse virtually all used contraception. Jewish congregations were not more or less likely than Christian congregations to have provided information on contraception. According to the survey responses of youth, Jewish parents were more likely than Christian parents to have provided that guidance to their teens. The Islamic youth were not likely to have received information on contraception from their congregations or their parents, but the numbers of those youth having intercourse were very low.

Youth from congregations which did supply information about contraception (about 8% of responding congregations) reported no instances of pregnancy. Youth from those congregations were not any more likely or less likely than other youth in the study to have had sexual intercourse. Thus it appears that the provision of information on contraception by the congregation does not make teens more likely to be sexually active but does give them protection if they are.

Being involved in a congregation gives no automatic protection against pregnancy, and it also gives no automatic protection against HIV and other sexually transmitted diseases. According to the National Survey of Adolescents and Young Adults: Sexual Health Knowledge, Attitudes, and Experiences study, one in four sexually active young people get a sexually transmitted disease each year. In that study, only 2% of the adolescents reported having contracted a sexually transmitted disease [Kaiser Family Foundation, 2003].

In our own study, 9% of those who were sexually active reported having contracted a sexually transmitted disease. It's difficult to know why a larger number of the teens in our study reported having gotten such a disease than teens reported in the other study. In both studies, the probability is that the actual number of teens with sexually transmitted diseases was higher than reported. It may be that the youth in our study were more aware that they had a sexually transmitted disease or were more willing to reveal that information on a survey which they personally placed in a mailbox. It's also possible that the youth in our study were less careful about disease prevention.

Practices and Attitudes about Contraception

We asked those teenagers who are having intercourse to share the kind of contraception they had used the most recent time. As shared earlier, 19.5% did not use any kind of contraception the most recent time. That is lower than the 27.4% who did not use contraception the first time they had intercourse, but it is still an alarmingly high figure. Condoms were the most commonly used, with 12.3% supplementing the condom with another form of contraception (most often the pill). Over half, 57.3%, did not use a condom, which is also an alarming figure with the risk of HIV and other sexually transmitted diseases. Here are the methods of contraception used for protection the most recent time:

30.4%	Condom
23.3%	Birth control pills
19.5%	None
12.3%	Condom plus another method
6.5%	Depo Provera or Norplant
4.3%	Other
3.7%	Withdrawal

The survey asked the teens whether or not they had all the information they needed about contraception. Among those teens who have had intercourse, only 61.9% agreed that they had all the information they need. Among teens who have not had intercourse, only 26.2% agreed that they had all the information they need. Here are some comments from teens about the use of contraception:

I know we should use condoms. I talked to my doctor and got Norplant, which was a good move. But we still need condoms for protection from disease. My boyfriend is like super ashamed to go into a store and buy them. I've kept saying that was his responsibility. I'm taking care of pregnancy prevention; his job is disease prevention. But he won't do it. I guess I'm going to have to get them. Female–Roman Catholic Church

Man, answering all these questions hurts me. It makes me see what a chance we're taking. We used a rubber the first time, but we haven't done anything the last three times. I didn't like the way the rubber felt, and I'm still not sure I put it on right. But that's no excuse. Male–Primitive Baptist Church

A doctor came to our youth group and talked to us about birth control. He told us how we could get it confidentially and why we should use a condom plus something else. I'm so thankful we got that information. I've been on the pill, and we always use a condom. It's the responsible thing to do. Female–United Church of Christ

My girlfriend says that she's the one who should take the major responsibility, because she would be the one who got pregnant. I suppose that's true, but I don't see that leaving me in the clear. I feel just as responsible as she does. If she got pregnant, I'd have an obligation to her and the baby. Male–Unitarian

I'm an airhead about most of my life, but not about being protected for sex. I love oral sex and intercourse, but I also know we're gambling with our futures when we do it. I take the pill, and I keep condoms in my purse. Female–United Methodist Church

I'm thankful that my girlfriend is on the pill. I would be embarrassed to buy condoms, but some of these questions make me wonder if it's a mistake not to be using a condom too. Male–Synagogue [Reformed]

The survey included some statements related to factual information about contraception and protection from HIV and other sexually transmitted diseases. The teens were asked to indicate whether each statement was true or false. **The figures which follow are the percentages of teens who answered each question correctly.** The correct factual answer is provided in parenthesis.

74%   The pill protects against HIV and other STDs. (False. It offers no protection against HIV and other STDs.)

66%   A woman can get a shot every three months that offers protection against pregnancy. (True. Depo Provera is a shot that is almost 100% effective at preventing pregnancy. Norplant, rods that are placed under the skin of the arm, is as effective and lasts at least three years. The failure rate for both of these is less than 1%.)

73%   Condoms fail too often to be worth using. (False. Correctly used, condoms work 95 to 98 percent of the time.)

87%   If you put a condom on incorrectly or use the wrong kind of lubricant with it, the condom will not be effective. (True. Because of this, the actual user effectiveness of condoms is 86% to 90% rather than the higher effectiveness which is possible.)

26%   There is no emergency contraception or "morning after" pill or pills that can prevent pregnancy. (False. Emergency contraception within 72 hours of unprotected sex can prevent pregnancy 72 to 75 percent of the time.)

76%   The pill isn't very effective in preventing pregnancy. (False. The pill, taken daily, is 95% to 97% effective.)

68%   The pill often has side effects that are fairly serious.
(False. The pill is very safe. It may even protect
against ovarian and uterine cancer. Some types of
the pill help acne. Most women do not gain weight
on the pill.)

On every factual item, females were more likely than males to choose the correct answer. Jewish and Unitarian Universalist youth were more likely than Christian youth to know the correct answers. With the exception of one category, those teens who have had intercourse were somewhat more likely than other teens to know the correct answers to the questions, but the magnitude of the difference was not reassuring. The exception came in those teens who had not used contraception at the time of their most recent intercourse–that group of teens showed even less knowledge about the factual aspects of birth control and protection against disease than was present in teens who are not yet having intercourse.

The survey also invited teens to respond to some items concerning attitudes about contraception and disease prevention. Here are the percentages of females and of males who agreed with each statement:

Talking about contraception and disease prevention before
having intercourse is a sign of respect for each other.
Females–90%   Males–81%

The girl and the guy should equally share responsibility
for contraception and disease prevention.
Females–91%   Males–78%

The girl has more influence than the guy on the kind
of contraception used.
Females–78%   Males–57%

I'd be embarrassed to go to a store and buy condoms.
Females–73%   Males–64%

Here are some of the comments made by teens concerning attitudes toward contraception and disease prevention:

I appreciated my boyfriend asking to talk about what kind of protection we should use. That shows he cares about me and cares about our future. Female–Evangelical Lutheran Church

Betty and I had so much trouble talking to each other about sex and birth control. We did just fine talking about other people having sex and about how stupid people were who got pregnant or got HIV. But it took us a long time to talk through our own relationship. Once we'd done it, we both felt better. We didn't want to hurt each other, and we didn't want to take any chances. Male–Disciples of Christ

If you left it up to the guy, none of them would use a rubber. My boyfriend keeps telling me how it would feel so much better not to have rubber between us. I tell him to think about how it would feel not to be having any sex. Female–American Baptist Church

Our youth leader had each of us sit across from a person of the opposite sex and maintain eye contact and say these words: oral sex, intercourse, clitoris, vagina, birth control pill, condom, and more. . . . At first we got red in the face and did this awkward laughing. Then it started to feel okay. It helped us feel that it was okay to talk about these things. If you're going to have sex with someone, you'd better talk about these things. Male–United Methodist Church

I had a boyfriend who told me that we didn't have to use a condom because we weren't having sex with anyone else and I was on the pill. I let him talk me out of it. Then I found out he'd been sleeping with my best friend as well as with me. With friends like the two of them, you don't need any enemies. Female–African Methodist Episcopal Church

My girlfriend and I had this deep, deep, deep talk about what it would mean to have sex with each other and about her getting on the pill and me getting condoms. By the time we talked about what we needed to do and how it would feel for her to go to the doctor for a prescription, we decided we weren't ready for sex. Male–Synagogue [Reformed]

A Challenge for Congregations

All of the adults who participated in this study, through surveys and through focus groups, had strong concerns about the welfare of the young people in their congregations and in their communities. The results of the study make it painfully clear to us that many young people connected with our congregations are not receiving the information which they need:

- to make healthy decisions about the kinds of sexual behaviors in which they will participate.

- to make healthy decisions about contraception and disease prevention if they are choosing to have oral sex and/or sexual intercourse.

We find ourselves deeply concerned about the amount of misinformation which some of these young people have on both contraception and disease prevention. Congregational involvement is important in the lives of virtually all the teens who participated in this study, and they are very receptive to more information and dialogue in congregational settings. It is a mistake for us to assume that they will receive adequate information from other sources and that our congregations have no responsibility in this area.

We should not assume that teens will obtain the information they need from schools, parents, friends, and the media. If we are truly concerned about youth in our faith communities, then we need to take the appropriate steps to see that they have the information they need to make healthy decisions about their sexuality, including contraception and disease prevention. Having that information does not make them more likely to have sexual intercourse, but it does make them less likely to become pregnant.

We had congregations participating in the study from traditions which are adamantly opposed to abortion under any circumstances and from traditions which affirm the right of a woman to have an abortion. Whether adults are pro-life or pro-choice, however, all who participated in the study would prefer that teens not become pregnant. Teens who are not pregnant do not have to make decisions about abortions.

It's a sobering fact to recognize that half the teens in our study who became pregnant chose to end that pregnancy with an abortion. It's even more sobering to realize this abortion rate appears to have been influenced in part by the perception that both families and congregations would have difficulty accepting the teen as unmarried and pregnant.

We strongly recommend:

- That congregations create settings and opportunities in which teens can talk about sexual matters and their relationship to the spiritual life.

- That congregations provide teens with the information that they need about abstinence and also about contraception and disease prevention. Comprehensive sexuality education belongs in our churches and other faith-based institutions.

- That all congregations provide classes for parents to equip them with the knowledge and skills needed to discuss these matters with their teens. Congregations which are not ready to do comprehensive sexuality education working directly with their youth can still take initiatives with parents.

- That clergy, youth teachers, and youth advisors receive the training they need to give solid, positive guidance to youth in these critical areas.

- That congregations affirm their love and respect for teenagers, regardless of what happens in the lives of those teens. Teenagers who become pregnant should feel that the congregation will be a supportive presence rather than a judgmental presence.

Chapter Five
Unwanted Sexual Experiences

*I can't exactly say that I was raped. He didn't use
physical force, and I didn't shove him away. But
I didn't want to do it. I kept explaining why I didn't
think I was ready. No matter what I said, he just
kept saying that if I loved him, I would do it with
him. We would go a little further each time, and
finally I let him push into me. I wish now that I'd
stopped him, but I couldn't make myself do it at
the time. He should have respected me more, and
I should have respected myself more.*

          Female
          Evangelical Lutheran

Social, Emotional, and Physical Force

Not all unwanted sexual experiences are the result of
physical force. In the study, we found that social pressure and
the desire to be accepted are more likely than physical force to be
responsible for a teenager being pushed into a sexual experience
in which he or she does not want to participate. The Evangelical
Lutheran teenager just quoted also had this to say:

*I don't know what is wrong with me. Why am I so afraid
to stand up for myself and to say firmly, "Stop that. Right
now"? Or better yet, before anything has happened, "Don't
you even think about it. We won't do that until I say it's
okay, and that day may not come with you." But I start to
feel like my whole world will fall apart if he rejects me,
so I give him this unhealthy power over me. I wish someone could help me stop it.*

Not surprisingly, females were more likely than males to
report having had unwanted sexual experiences. Females were
also more likely than males to express a desire for programs to
help them be more assertive and for programs on how to avoid
rape, sexual harassment, and sexual abuse. In one of our focus

groups, a female minister and mother of two teenagers shared this observation:

> *In this culture, there are still big differences between males and females in assertiveness about sex. Guys are much more inclined to ask for and push for what they want, and girls are more likely to feel that they need to nurture and please. I still don't feel like I can say "No" to my husband when he wants to do something sexually, but he says "No" to me with some frequency.*

Several other persons in focus groups commented on the reality that our culture encourages males to be more assertive or even aggressive and females to be "nice." In sexual relationships, that can have tragic consequences. Among 11th and 12th graders, we found that females were more than twice as likely as males to have had unwanted sexual experiences.

Have you ever had an unwanted sexual experience?

	9th-10th Grades	11th-12th Grades
Male	6%	12%
Female	12%	31%

We asked those who reported such experiences to indicate how the pressure for the unwanted experience came:

Primarily physical pressure	12%
Primarily social or emotional pressure	76%
Uncertain	12%

Even when teens checked primarily physical pressure, they almost always indicated that social or emotional pressure was also strongly involved. The pressure can take many forms and sometimes reflects the perceived expectations which are present in the school. Consider this teenage girl's experience:

> *There's like this unwritten policy in my school that if you go out with somebody three times that on the fourth time you're supposed to put out. I stopped dating two different boys because of that. Then I started going out with a boy that I thought was very nice, and I didn't think he would be that way. But he was. I fought him enough that he didn't make me have regular sex, but I had to give him oral sex to get*

*him to let me up. . . . No one talks about this kind of thing. No
one does at school. No one does at church. I live with Mom,
and she doesn't have any idea what goes on in my life.*

Physical force placed a role, but she recognized that the
"unwritten rule" in her school played a factor in what happened
to her. Such expectations can make life difficult for both males
and females. An 11th grade male commented:

*Beth and I have been a couple since we started high school,
and I really love her. We agreed that we weren't going to
have sex. Jesus is important to both of us, and we don't want
to do something we think is wrong. I hurt Beth really bad
because of something I didn't say. The fellows on the
basketball team are always talking about who they're
having sex with. Who gives great head. And some of them
kept pushing, wanting me to say what Beth and I were
doing. By refusing to answer a question one day, I ended
up giving the impression that Beth and I have slept together.
Then one of these a - - - - - - buddies of mine told his sister who
told Beth. Beth was so hurt. I left the team. I wasn't going
to let myself be put in that kind of situation again.*

A 12th grade male shared this perspective:

*Some of the fellows I hang with talk like sex is this impersonal
thing that you do–like the girl is just an object instead of a
person. And they talk like the goal is to do as much as you
can, whether the other person wants to do it or not. Some of
the talk is just crap. People haven't really done everything
they claim they have. But some have. And when I'm with
them, I start to feel like there's something wrong with me
because I haven't had sex yet. But the problem isn't with me.
The problem is with them.*

The teens in one of the groups in which we talked about the
survey results had a very animated discussion about the impact
of peer expectations on what couples do when they are together.
The girls in the group talked about the tension between getting a
reputation of being "cheap" and getting the reputation of
"thinking you're better than everybody else." Those who get the
reputation of being "cheap" are seen as far too ready to have sex
and are not respected by others. On the other hand, those who
appear not to be having intercourse or oral sex can be seen as

thinking they are better than other people. Most of the teens in the group didn't want to be viewed by others as being in either of those categories.

The boys in the group agreed that there were certain girls who were viewed as being "easy." While fellows might go out with girls they viewed in that way and attempt to take advantage of them, they tended not to have respect for them. They also agreed that some girls were seen as being cold and that those girls were sometimes referred to as "uptight bitches." The boys in the group acknowledged that the older you were, the greater the pressure was on you to have had sexual intercourse. Several fellows felt that others would eventually start to act like there was something wrong with you if you didn't talk like you'd had intercourse or at least oral sex.

Those peer expectations create a climate in which young people can feel under pressure to have intercourse and oral sex. That pressure can cause males to be more aggressive and can cause females to be less forceful in resisting. A male parent in one of the focus groups where we talked about the results made this observation:

> *In some ways our society has made a lot of progress in male and female roles in the workplace. But it seems to me that we've made less in dating and sex. When I was in high school, the general expectation was that guys were looking to have sex and girls were being careful about giving it up. I'm not sure that we've moved very far beyond those stereotypes.*

And to some extent that parent is right. We haven't moved as far beyond those stereotypes as one would like—not in the face of 31% of teenage girls in the 11th and 12th grades having had unwanted sexual experiences. Yet not all of the aggressiveness is on the part of males. Here are some comments from teenage males:

> *I was surprised to find out how much more experienced my girlfriend was. It's like she had done everything, and I'd done almost nothing. I made a fool out of myself trying to act like I knew more than I did. And we did some things that I wasn't ready for.* Junior–United Methodist Church

*I'm not sure how I feel about oral sex. There's something
about it that makes me feel used. I don't like the taste,
and I can never seem to get in a comfortable position. My
girlfriend absolutely refuses to give me oral sex. She says
it makes her feel degraded. But she wants it from me. I
don't want her to lose interest in me, so I go along with it.
It's not okay for her to be degraded, but it's okay for me to
be.* Sophomore–Evangelical Covenant Church

Several of the Muslim youth indicated that they feel trapped
between two worlds. Their families expect that their youth will
have no sexual experiences before marriage and actively discourage or prohibit dating. That expectation is especially strong on
Muslim females. Yet most of the Muslim youth in our study
attended schools with large numbers of non-Muslim youth.
While fewer Muslim females dated than any other religious group
in the study, those who did were more likely than their Christian
and Jewish peers to report having had unwanted sexual
experiences. From the comments which they made, it appears
that this was primarily the case when they were dating non-
Muslim youth. Muslim males who dated were not any more or
less likely than their Christian and Jewish peers to report
unwanted sexual experiences.

Alcohol, Drugs, Love, and Rape

In responding to the first survey item on "unwanted sexual
experiences," respondents defined for themselves what constituted such an experience. Another item asked them to be more
specific in describing those experiences. The total is more than
100% for females. Many respondents had more than one type of
unwanted experience:

Unwanted Activity	Males	Females
Unwanted sexual intercourse	2%	11%
Unwanted oral sex	11%	38%
Unwanted touching below the waist	15%	53%
Unwanted touching above the waist	10%	68%
Unwanted kissing	35%	62%
Other unwanted experiences	16%	19%

Of those females who had experienced unwanted sexual
intercourse, almost exactly half felt that they had been raped.

The others felt that they had been pushed into intercourse but did not want to describe what had happened as rape. In comments from youth on the survey itself and in interviews, these reasons were shared for not wanting to call the unwanted sexual intercourse rape:

- Some felt that it was not rape if they had not been physically forced to have intercourse. If the pressure was entirely social or emotional, they did not feel it had been rape.

- Some did not feel it was rape because they knew the person who was responsible for the unwanted experience. Those teens felt that "rape" is something that is done to you by a stranger. Very few teens had their unwanted experiences, of any kind, with strangers.

- Some indicated that they did not want to define themselves as "rape victims." They felt better about themselves if they accepted some responsibility for the unwanted experience.

None of the males who indicated having had unwanted sexual intercourse felt they had been raped.

The number of teens who indicated that they had been personally responsible for the unwanted sexual experience of another person was less than a fourth the number who reported having such unwanted experiences. There are several possible explanations for the gap between those who had been victims and those who acknowledged that they had been aggressors:

- It is possible that the teens who participated in this study were less likely than other teens to have been responsible for inflicting unwanted experiences on others. That is the explanation which those of us who are active in faith-based institutions would most like to be true.

- A teen who is sexually aggressive may well be responsible for the unwanted experiences of more than one other young person.

- Some teens may in fact fail to recognize the extent to which, through emotional or social pressure, they forced others to do something they did not want.

- Some teens may simply have been unwilling to take responsibility for their actions by admitting them even on an anonymous survey. It may have been personally too painful to do so. In spite of our best efforts to reassure teens of anonymity, it's also possible some were afraid the responses would be traced back to them.

Comments from some teens acknowledged that it had been very difficult for them to come to see themselves as having taken advantage of another person. For example:

I screwed up. When my girl friend and I were together, I honestly thought she was okay about everything we did. Sometimes she'd say no or push at me, but it always seemed kind of playful to me, like she was into it. When she broke up with me, she told me that I didn't respect her body and that meant I didn't respect her. At first I didn't agree. I sure never intended to pressure her. But then I started to see that I should never have gone ahead when she said no. Male–Presbyterian Church

The worst moment of my life was when my girl friend and her mother came to our home to talk with my parents and with me. I could tell they were pissed from the moment they came in the door. My girl friend thought I had tried to rape her. I didn't see it that way at all, but by the time she was done talking and crying I did. If they had gone to the police, my life would have been over. And I would have had it coming. I look back now and have trouble believing what I did. Male–African Methodist Episcopal Church

Bob was two years younger than me. He was such a hunk and had gone out with enough people that I thought he was sexually experienced. I was wrong, and I handled it all wrong. I made him feel inadequate and then made him feel like he had to do what I wanted. I made too many assumptions, and we didn't talk about things. Female–Synagogue [Reformed]

While force played a role, particularly in those instances when the unwanted sexual experience was intercourse, the social and emotional pressure and horrible lack of communication were greater factors. Several factors were very clear among the teens in our study who were a part of unwanted sexual experiences:

- Some still do not accept the concept that "No means no." There is a tremendous tendency, especially in the midst of strong sexual arousal, to ignore clear requests for activities to stop.

- Some, particularly females, have not learned to say "No" with force and conviction–ideally before sexual exploration has begun. Often "maybes" or unclear messages are given.

- Most teens have not talked together about what they do and do not want to do sexually. The sharing of affection and exploration begins, and whatever communication takes place is under very difficult circumstances.

- The desire to be accepted and loved is a major factor in some teens going further than they really want sexually. There is also a double standard at work. Boys are "supposed to" try to go further, and girls are "supposed to" stop them.

- Some of the written comments suggest that there are some "unwanted experiences" which only become unwanted later–when the sexual activity doesn't result in the relationship for which one of the participants had hoped.

Alcohol and drugs also play a significant role in unwanted sexual experiences. Among the teens in the study who had unwanted sexual experiences, 26.3% indicated that they were using alcohol or drugs on at least one of the occasions when they had such an experience. A 2001 Kaiser Family Foundation study on 1200 secular teens found that 29% did more sexually than they had planned because alcohol or drugs constituted part of the situation.

In our study, alcohol was three times more likely to be a factor than any illegal drug. In written comments and in interviews, teens talked about the significant extent to which alcohol and drugs lowered inhibitions. For example:

When I drink, I become like this totally different person. Nothing seems like a big deal, and I just want to have fun. I should never drink when I'm with a guy. Female–United Methodist

I like to drink when I'm with a girl because it helps me not be so nervous. When I'm sober, I'm this shy, up-tight little boy. When I drink, I have more confidence in myself and feel like an adult. . . . The only problem is that I also lose my self-control. I've done things when I'm drunk that I'd never do sober. Male–Southern Baptist

A very candid teen in a youth group meeting made the interesting observation that she doesn't get drunk on alcohol but gets "drunk on love." She explained that she wants so much to feel that she's loved that she'll do things she would not under other circumstances. "If a boy knows enough to tell me that he loves me, then he's found the key to my heart and the key to my panties. I don't like it, but that's how I am." She said it with humor, and the group gave her an embarrassed laugh in response. The humor, however, was a mask for a very serious issue, and subsequent discussion in the group showed that she was not the only one who felt that way.

The desire for approval; the desire for love; pressure from friends; alcohol and drugs; and poor communication are all factors which can make teen more vulnerable to unwanted sexual experiences. Tragically parents, schools, and faith-based institutions have not done enough to make teens aware of these factors and to prepare them for healthier decision-making.

Unwanted Sexual Experiences with Adults and Family

Not all the unwanted experiences were with other teenagers. Females who were in dating relationships with older males who were out of high school were 31% more likely to have had intercourse than those dating males in high school–and they were 21% more likely to have had unwanted sexual experiences.

Thus the study gives reinforcement to the common parental concern about high school age females dating older males. The older males are likely to be more sexually experienced and to be more assertive in what they want. (The number of high school males dating older females who were out of high school was too small for any conclusions to be drawn.) An 11th grade Presbyterian female shares these observations about the dating relationship she had as a 10th grader with a male who was a college sophomore:

> *I have a father who's eight years older than my mother, and I threw that up to them when they complained about my dating someone four years older. But now that I look back, I see that it was a mistake. Four years may not mean that much when you're thirty, but it means a lot when you're sixteen. Until he went to college, John just lived down the street from us; and I guess I had a crush on him most of my life. When he asked me to go to a movie with him when he was home on summer break, it was like a dream come true. My parents weren't going to let me go with him, but we both told them it was just a friendship thing, so they let me. Then we just kept moving ahead in small stages until he was coming home every weekend to have time with me. And I'd go visit him on campus–lying to my folks and saying I was staying with a girl there when I was with him.*

> *He knew so much more about sex than I did. I felt uncomfortable at the time with some of the things we did, but I wanted so desperately to come across as mature that I went along with anything he wanted. Of course I see that clearly now in a way that I didn't at the time.*

> *The biggest price was that I started living in his college world in my mind more than in high school. I started viewing my high school friends as immature and had no interest at all in the high school boys. I was pretty cruel to some people, and I'm amazed they are still. . . friends.*

The perspective which she gained on the problems of dating someone who was in college only became clear to her after the relationship ended. Most of the high school girls in the study who were currently dating males who were out of high school did not share that kind of self-awareness, even if they had gone through unwanted sexual experiences.

Some of the worst unwanted experiences which were reported involved adults who were much older than the teens and generally in some kind of family relationship. This very graphic account from an 11th grade female is particularly disturbing because of the failure of a pastor to offer help to the teen:

My stepfather makes me suck his d - - - after school two or three days a week. I talked to my mother about it, and she said I was lying. Then I told her about it right in front of him. He denied it completely and said I was probably making it up because he was too busy and didn't give me much attention. . . .

Then I talked about it to our pastor. He talked to my parents, and he believed my stepfather rather than me. They don't believe that this is happening. . . . He [the stepfather] was very angry when I talked to my mother in front of him. Then the pastor talking to him earned me a . . . beating. The bastard said he'd put my mother in the hospital if I ever told anyone again. So I keep on doing it and letting them act like they are so religious. I'd like to bite it off, but I don't have the guts.

We failed to ask a specific question in the study about sexual experiences with family members, so our results are limited to the comments teens made in describing unwanted sexual experiences or to experiences shared in interviews. We had reports of unwanted sexual experiences with fathers, stepfathers, stepmothers, brothers, sisters, stepbrothers, and stepsisters. We did not have any reports of unwanted experiences with mothers. This account from a 12th grade male shares considerable conflict about his relationship with a stepsister:

My stepsister and I have been having sex with each other every chance we get for the last two years. It's a huge secret. Absolutely no one knows about it. We're very careful, and we both go out with other people.

The first time happened because she was flirting with me, and I responded more strongly than she expected. I ended up partly undressing her. She asked me not to do it, but I thought she was still kidding. . . . It was only later

*that I realized I'd pushed too hard. Nothing happened
for about two months after that, and I spent every day
scared out of my mind that she would tell her mother
or my father. That would have been such a disaster.
Then she really turned the tables on me. She threatened
to tell them if I didn't do what she wanted me to do. The
difference was that I was really, really, really willing to
do anything she wanted.*

*So it started with her flirting. Then I forced her. Then
she forced me. But there's no force going on now. We
both want it. The question is what we do when we are
both out of high school. If our parents hadn't married,
there would be nothing wrong with our dating or even
marrying each other. Maybe there still isn't, but I don't
think most people could handle it. I'm not sure the two
of us could handle anyone knowing about this.*

The most frequently reported unwanted sexual experiences
with family members involved girls and their stepfathers. Those
incidents were much more frequently reported than any
involving biological fathers. The inhibitions which are present in
the biological relationship seem, at least among those teens who
shared experiences with us, not to be as strong between
stepfathers and stepdaughters. What was particularly alarming
to us as we read the accounts was that several of these
situations were ongoing, and the teen was not talking about it
with a parent or any other adult. Those teens who indicated
that they had reported the experience and that it had stopped
had most frequently talked to a parent other than the offender
or in some instances to a youth pastor. They were more likely to
report having visited with a youth pastor than with any other
adult outside of the family. While these are anecdotal reports
rather than hard statistics, they do reinforce the value of youth
pastors having positive relationships with teens. They can
become "the safe place" to share painful experiences.

Prevention

What can we do to prevent unwanted sexual experiences for our teens? We'll have more to say about this in future chapters on programming in faith-based institutions, but some observations are important within the context of this chapter:

- Teens need help examining male and female gender roles and the expectations peers place on males and females. They need to question the aggressiveness associated with males and the more submissive nature associated with females.

- Teens need help in thinking through their sexual values and determining for themselves how far they want to go sexually. They need to develop those values and determinations out of their own faith, healthy knowledge about sexuality, understanding the values of their parents, and recognizing their own goals for the future.

- Teens need help developing communication skills and gaining comfort talking about sexuality with potential partners—at times when they are not sexually aroused. Both males and females need to be comfortable saying "yes" and "no" to sexual activities.

- Teens need to develop healthy assertiveness and adequate self-confidence to stand up for themselves.

- Teens need to learn the roles that alcohol, drugs, and social and emotional pressure can play in sexual decisions and behavior.

- Teens need to learn that respecting the right of another person to say no is part of having a healthy relationship. They also need to learn that physical force is never appropriate in a sexual relationship or in any other relationship.

Equal Dating

We visited with youth in five congregational settings about ways in which dating relationships could be improved. The concept of "equal dating" was an attractive one to the teens in those settings. They suggested that equal dating could be described in this way:

1. In equal dating, either person is free to ask the other out or to suggest an activity. A male doesn't have to take the responsibility all the time, and a female can take the initiative.
2. In equal dating, communication is encouraged, and impression-making is not needed. Couples discuss and plan their activities together. Their goal will be to help each other have a good time rather than one trying to impress the other.
3. In equal dating, financial responsibilities are shared. Specifics with this may vary depending on who has more money, but the general goal is for both parties to participate in the cost of activities. Then no one "owes" the other anything. If there is a kiss at the end of the date, it's because both people want to do it–not because one person bought dinner.
4. In equal dating, the couple "owns" the relationship together. The couple works to be honest and to make caring decisions together. The relationship continues only if both want it to do so.
5. In equal dating, each person has a right to be an individual. He or she has a right to time alone and with other people. Each has the right to change his or her mind and to be different than he or she was in the past.
6. In equal dating, each person has the responsibility to be kind. Doors are opened by the one who reaches them first, and no one assumes that he or she has certain privileges or rights because of being male or female.
7. In equal dating, sexual decision-making is a mutual task with clear communication. Unless both persons want to do something, it doesn't happen.

Chapter Six
Gay, Lesbian, and Bisexual Youth

*I never thought before about the possibility that we
actually had homosexual teenagers who were active
in our church. But with a youth group with forty
kids in it, we have to have some who are homosexual
or at least who are struggling with identity issues.
As negative as I've been about homosexuality, none
of them would ever approach me. That has to change.
We've got to find some more compassionate ways to
respond to these young people.*

Missouri Synod Lutheran Pastor

Tensions in the Faith Community

Homosexuality is a topic about which people of equally
strong faith are not always in agreement. Many denominations
have continuing internal debate about whether or not homosexuality is a sin and about issues of membership, ordination,
and unions for persons of homosexual orientation or behavior.
Some long-time members of faith communities have changed to
different religious traditions because of denominational or
congregational positions on homosexuality.

In our focus group discussions prior to the actual survey
process and in our discussion groups about the survey data, we
heard spirited discussions surrounding questions like these:

- Is homosexuality a sin?

- Is there a genetic basis or reason for homosexuality?

- Can people who are homosexual really be "converted"
  to a heterosexual orientation?

- What should the faith community be doing to respond
  to the prejudice against homosexual persons which
  exists in the larger society?

- Should the matter of sexual orientation or behavior be a factor in determining membership in a faith-based community?

- Should the matter of sexual orientation or behavior be a factor in deciding to ordain a person for congregational leadership?

- Should a distinction be drawn between those persons who have a homosexual orientation but choose to remain celibate and those who engage in same sex sexual behaviors?

The topic of bisexuality drew considerable debate as well. Persons of both homosexual and heterosexual orientation frequently had problems with the concept of bisexuality. Some persons in focus groups talked about bisexuality as a "stage" that people go through before realizing that their "true" orientation is homosexual. Some expressed agreement with the concept that homosexuality and heterosexuality are in fact on a continuum with bisexuality the middle ground and that people may be found anywhere along that continuum.

When we reviewed sexuality education literature from many denominational traditions, we observed that:

- There are a few denominations in which homosexuality is accepted as fully as heterosexuality and in no way viewed as a sin. Those traditions reflect that in their resources.

- There are many denominations in which the official position is that homosexuality is a sin but in which a distinction is made between those of homosexual orientation and of homosexual behavior. Acceptance is extended to those of homosexual orientation who are celibate but not to those who are actively involved in a homosexual relationship.

- There are denominations in which homosexuality is viewed as a sin and in which there is a firm belief that people of that orientation can be converted or changed to a heterosexual orientation.

- There are some denominations in which the existing sexuality education resources reflect the kind of confusion and conflict over the issue that is present in the denomination. For example, some of those resources speak about the importance of accepting persons of homosexual orientation and maintain that such orientation is not simply a matter of "choice." Homosexuality is not seen as a barrier to membership. But those same traditions then talk about it being impossible to be homosexual and be ordained. If the orientation and behavior are not sinful, why is ordination prohibited?

In virtually all of the religious sexuality education resources that we reviewed, with the exception of the first category above, the discussion seems to assume that homosexual persons are not active in the youth class or group–they are outside in the community. Thus even materials which are very accepting of homosexuality as an orientation often appear to take it for granted that there are no young people of homosexual orientation participating in the study. (The *Our Whole Lives* curriculum from the Unitarian Universalist Association and the United Church Board for Homeland Ministries is an exception.)

Surprising Percentages

If we had a preconceived idea of what we would find about the sexual orientation of teens who were involved in faith-based institutions, it was that we would likely discover a smaller percentage of teens self-identifying as homosexual or bisexual than has been found in secular studies. Our assumption was that teens of homosexual or bisexual orientation would be somewhat less likely to be involved in a faith-based institution, given the number of traditions with a negative view of homosexuality.

In looking at our results, it's important to be aware that forming a sexual identity is a developmental task of the adolescent years. Some sexuality education professionals report that as many as 25% of twelve year olds are unsure of their sexual orientation but that only 5% of eighteen year olds have that same uncertainty.

What we found, in fact, was that a surprisingly high number of teenagers who are involved in faith-based institutions self-identified as homosexual or bisexual. In fact some secular studies have reported lower percentages of teens with homosexual or bisexual orientation than we found. As we have shared the results with clergy and other congregational leaders, most have been surprised by the percentage of teens who didn't have a heterosexual orientation. Remember that these figures reflect self-identification of orientation, not behavior:

	Males	Females
Heterosexual	86%	89%
Homosexual	7%	5%
Bisexual	5%	4%
Don't know	2%	2%

Some of our most extensive written comments came from youth who self-identify as homosexual or bisexual and who have anxiety both about how to relate their sexual orientation to their faith and about how accepted they would be if their sexual orientation were known by the congregation. For example:

I'm about as deep in the closet as a homosexual can be. My parents don't know. No one in my youth group knows. Almost no one at school knows. This other guy and I have been good friends since second grade. When we were in the fifth grade, we started touching each other. Then we started to do other things and liked it. . . . Neither one of us is all that attracted to girls. We're careful not to hang out with each other too much at school. And fortunately our parents don't think anything about our spending time together in our rooms because we've always been friends. . . . Both of us are thinking we should ask girls to the prom. It isn't exactly fair to them in one way, but we'd probably be asking people who wouldn't get to go if not with us. . . . Kids at church and our youth advisor make these jokes about fags and queers. I'd never be accepted there if they knew I was gay. Junior–Southern Baptist Church

The only person in my synagogue who knows I'm bisexual is the girl that started doing things with me. . . . I think our rabbi believes that Jewish people are never homosexual–that it's like a condition that only Gentiles can get. . . . I just took for

granted that I was a heterosexual when I was in middle school and a freshman. I dated and made out, and I loved doing that . . . . Then this friend and I were staying overnight, and we started talking about how the guys we dated didn't know how to touch you right. And we started doing things to each other, and it was great. I still like guys too, but it isn't possible for me to have as much pleasure with a guy as with her. . . . I think that many people have a homosexual side to them, but they bury it because society disapproves. . . . I can't decide whether God cares about my being bi. Senior–Synagogue [Reformed]

Secret Lives

The majority of these teens have not been open with clergy or other adult leaders about their sexual orientation. Eighty-eight percent of the teens who self-identified as homosexual or bisexual indicated that their pastor (or other cleric) was not aware of their orientation. Only 36% indicated that there was a youth worker, advisor, or other adult leader (besides a parent) in the church who was aware of their orientation.

Most of these teens do have at least one young person in the faith-based institution who knows about their orientation, so they are not completely isolated. Eighty-three percent indicated that there was at least one young person in the faith-based institution who was aware of their orientation, but only 16% said that the whole youth group or class knew about it. Very few of them have felt sufficiently comfortable to "come out" to their entire youth group or class.

Almost half of these youth (46%) said that their parents were not aware of their sexual orientation or of their struggle over identifying their sexual orientation. The authors of this book were deeply concerned as we went through survey responses and as we interviewed teens of homosexual or bisexual orientation to discover how many of them are leading secret lives–at least in their homes and in their faith-based institutions. Sexual orientation is a basic part of our identity, and we feel it is a significant problem when teens are not able to comfortably talk about such concerns with their parents and in their faith-based institutions.

Non-heterosexual teens in our study were almost twice as likely as heterosexual teens to have seriously considered suicide. This should be a matter of significant concern for those of us in faith-based institutions.

If the teens perceived that their pastor or another adult in the church felt "open, accepting, or nonjudgmental" about matters of sexual orientation, they were much more likely to have talked with someone in the congregation about the topic. Here are some comments about adult leaders and congregational youth groups from teens with a homosexual, bisexual, or undetermined sexual orientation:

We have a great youth pastor. He always says that we can talk to him about anything, and he means it. I started talking to him last year because I was starting to realize that I was gay and didn't know what to do about it. Some friends at school already suspected that I was gay and were starting to make comments. . . . He was completely accepting. He told me that he felt like homosexual behavior was a sin but that he didn't think you could choose whether or not you had homosexual feelings. . . . He's kept talking with me and has struggled to understand what I'm going through. I think some of his own opinions have been changed through talking to me. He gave me the courage to talk to my parents about this, and then he encouraged them to be supportive of me. I don't know what I would have done without him.
Junior–Independent Christian Church

There is no way I can be open in my church about being lesbian. Our pastor has preached sermons on the sin of homosexuality and on the danger of having homosexuals as teachers in school and in any kind of church leadership. The others in the youth group say nasty things about the kids at school they think are gay. I just keep my mouth shut. . . . I don't want to be lesbian. That's just the way I am. God had something to do with this, and I don't think God feels the same way the church does.
Sophomore–Nazarene Church

My minister is a strong advocate of rights for gay and lesbian people. He doesn't think being gay is a sin, and he's very open. . . . I talked with him a year ago when I was trying to figure out whether I was heterosexual or homosexual. . . . Then just a few weeks ago, I kind of came out to the youth group. I say kind of came out because it turns out that at least half of them already thought I was probably gay. The whole group was very supportive to me, and it was like a gigantic relief to not be hiding part of myself from them. I wish that kids at school would be as accepting. Sophomore–United Church of Christ

I've talked with my pastor about my being gay, and he's done his best to help me. He doesn't think being gay is this big sin, but he also says that life is sure a lot easier if you're heterosexual. He's encouraged me not to be in a hurry to call myself gay. . . . The thing is, I just think I am gay. I can't do anything about it. Anyway, he's really kind even though he hopes I don't "stay" like this. Freshman–United Methodist Church

My pastor helped my parents get me in this program that is supposed to make you into a heterosexual. I was in this small group with four others from different churches. We kept getting yelled at and prayed for and made to sign commitment cards about not doing any homosexual acts. At first I resented it. Then I thought that maybe they were right. I mean, gay isn't normal. That isn't what most people are. But I still find myself attracted to other guys rather than to girls. What am I supposed to do? I hate being this way. I know the pastor and my parents and the drill sergeant guy all want to help me, but I don't think they understand. I'm trying to figure out for myself if God understands. Junior–Independent Christian Church

We had extensive written comments from young people who see themselves as gay, lesbian, bisexual, or uncertain. We also interviewed some youth who were open with us about having a non-heterosexual orientation. The quotes shared in this chapter represent a very small percentage of the comments we have read and heard. It's very clear to us that almost none of the teens in the study who see themselves as homosexual or bisexual are "choosing" that orientation. Many of them readily acknowledge that it would be easier to be heterosexual and that they would like to be heterosexual because that is more accepted. Yet they find themselves with a non-heterosexual orientation or struggling with orientation issues.

Those youth who are non-heterosexual and who have a clergy person, youth group advisor, or youth group who are open and nonjudgmental are far more likely to be open within the faith-based community about their orientation. Those who were able to be open in their faith-based communities were also less likely to have considered suicide than other non-heterosexual teens in this study. Those who are in faith-based institutions where there are negative views toward homosexuality and bisexuality rarely are open about their orientation. Those teens live with a very painful silence.

In our focus groups, clergy and adult leaders from traditions which disapprove of homosexuality were struck by the high percentage of teens in this study who have non-heterosexual orientation. Almost all of them acknowledged the importance of being more open so that these teens can talk about issues of orientation in religious settings. Having that kind of openness, however, is very difficult when people genuinely believe that homosexuality is a sin. One African Episcopal Methodist pastor shared the dilemma in this way:

> *I am very sorry that I came here tonight, and I am very glad that I came here tonight. I am sorry because my life would have been a lot simpler without learning these things. We have a big youth group. And what I hear you saying is that we've got to have some gay and lesbian kids in that group. I'm glad I came because I can see that we need to do something about this. I think homosexual behavior is a sin, but it's clear that these kids aren't choose their homosexual orientation. So what do we want them to do? Be celibate forever? Become heterosexuals? I mean, their becoming heterosexual would be the solution for the church, but is that possible? . . . We simply have to find ways to talk with these kids. We've got to let them know that we don't blame them for an orientation and that God loves them and wants to help them. But how do we convey that when we see the behavior as a sin?*

Pastors of predominantly black congregations were more likely to disapprove of homosexual behavior than pastors in congregations with other ethnic compositions. The youth in those congregations were also more likely to indicate that their congregation disapproved of homosexual behavior. Black clergy in our focus groups said that they felt it was even more difficult to talk about homosexuality in a black congregation than in a white congregation and that it was difficult to talk about any sexually related topic in their churches.

A pastor in the United Methodist Church shared a very interesting perspective:

> *Think about what it says that there are so many kids in our churches who are gay and who aren't open about it. If I were gay and felt disapproval from the church, I'd stop coming. But most of these young people are continuing to be active. That says to me that God and the church are very important to them.*

The Faith-Based Institution Is Important

The United Methodist pastor was absolutely right. Religious faith and involvement in faith-based institutions are very important for the young people in this study who have a non-heterosexual orientation. We found no differences between heterosexual and non-heterosexual teens in the importance they placed on religion in their lives, on their commitment to God, on their frequency of prayer, or on their commitment to the faith-based institution.

The extensive written comments from non-heterosexual teenagers did make clear, however, that many of them struggle with their sexual orientation in relationship to their faith. For example:

> *I am so thankful that my pastor and church are not down on gay and lesbian people. My youth pastor sees being gay as another example of the diversity in people. I feel like everyone in the church is very accepting of me. But I feel sorry for some of my gay friends who are in churches that do not feel that way. I couldn't keep going to church if everyone disapproved of me.* Male–United Church of Christ

> *I can't be open with my parents or my church about being gay. They see being homosexual as sinful. . . . . I don't agree with them. I don't think that's how God sees me.*

101

God made me this way, and I don't think it was a mistake.
Female–Southern Baptist Church

*For a long time, I accepted what my church teaches. It's
not your fault if you have homosexual desires, but it is your
fault if you act on them. I'm not so sure that's right now.
Would God give you the desire, the feelings, if it was
wrong to act on them? Heterosexual people act on them.
I know I'm not ready for sex yet, but I will be in time. The
possibility of sex with a man has no appeal to me at all.
I'm not so sure that homosexual behavior is a sin.* Female–
Roman Catholic Church

*I'm in this constant state of torment over my sexuality.
I know that my church disapproves of being gay. I've
read the Bible and know there are verses that are against
homosexual behavior. But Jesus didn't preach a sermon
on sex. I don't see that the Bible makes homosexuality
into this huge sin. But I respect our pastor and youth
teacher. Maybe I'm wrong. Maybe it is a huge sin.
Then what I have to do is not have sex in order to stay
out of sin. I would like to talk to somebody about this,
but I don't want to become hated by people I like. Maybe
I'll give you people a call.* Male–Missouri Synod Lutheran
Church

That teen actually did give us a call. We had provided our
phone number with the surveys so that people with questions
could call us directly if they wished. We had a series of phone
conversations with this young person. He was very sincere in
his efforts to sort out the teachings of his church, his own
perceived sexual orientation, and his own beliefs about God.

Many of these teens are aware of religious teachings that
homosexual behavior is a sin but are not in agreement with
those teachings. The resulting internal struggle is a difficult one
for those teens to whom involvement in their faith-based
institutions is very important. Many religious traditions, as
already shared, are unclear about their positions on
homosexuality. Teens in those traditions pick up on that
uncertainty:

*My church is confused. It's okay to be homosexual and
be a member of the church. But you can't be homosexual*

and be a minister. *Why is that? I do not understand.*
I don't want to be a minister, so I should see it as a non-
issue for me. Male–Presbyterian Church U.S.A.

My father is the minister of our church. He goes to Annual
Conference every year, and every year there's debate
about something having to do with homosexuality. Dad has
changed his views on this since I worked up the nerve to
tell him that I was probably bisexual or a lesbian. He's
bought books about the Bible and theology that explain the
context of what the Bible says about sexual orientation.
Our denomination doesn't know what it believes on this
topic. You aren't supposed to be gay and be a minister,
but Dad knows several clergy who are gay. They just
don't announce it, and the bishop overlooks it. Dad says
most clergy would have a more accepting view if they
weren't afraid of losing financial support from conservatives
in the church. Female–United Methodist Church

Whatever the official position of the church on homosexual orientation and behavior, it is extremely important to remain aware of the teens in local congregations who do feel they have a non-heterosexual orientation and for whom the faith-based institution is extremely important.

Knowing People Who Are Gay

Ninety-six percent of the teens who completed surveys for this study indicate that they know at least one person their age (or within two years of their age) who has a gay, lesbian, or bisexual orientation. Most know several such persons. The 4% who indicated that they do not tended to be in more rural areas. While many teens who have such an orientation are reluctant to share that in their congregation much further than with one or two especially close friends, almost all teens know someone their age who is gay, lesbian, or bisexual. This is a part of life for teenagers today, and it is a part of life which the church needs to recognize.

We did not ask teens on the survey if they were open at school about being gay, lesbian, or bisexual. Based on the written comments of teens on the survey and on our interviews with teens, it appears to us:

- That religious teens are somewhat more likely to be open about a non-heterosexual orientation with more people at school than in the congregation.

- That there are some schools in which it is acceptable for non-heterosexual teens to be open about their orientation, and there are some schools in which it is very unacceptable.

- That even in the most accepting school settings, teens who are open about a gay, lesbian, or bisexual orientation can become the objects of ridicule, resentment, and derision.

We had extensive written comments from gay, lesbian, and bisexual teens on the dangers of being open about their orientation at school. While some of them choose to do so, the price can be very high. Some heterosexual teens in the study shared insights about justice and homosexuality:

My friend Beth is lesbian. I'd known that she was for maybe a year before she worked up the courage to tell me. It's fine with me that she is. But as she's started to be more open about it, life has gotten harder for her. I'm deeply offended by the comments and disgusting jokes that are made at school about gay and lesbian people. . . . Our pastor talked in a sermon about the importance of standing up for what you think is right. That made me realize that I need to take a clearer stand for the rights of people like Beth. I shouldn't just keep my mouth shut when people make ugly comments. Christ would have come to the defense of people being treated that way. Female–United Methodist Church

The Golden Rule tells us to do unto others like we would want them to be to us. But that's not what happens in our relationships with gay people at school. Some of my friends from church think there's nothing wrong with putting down the f - - -. I don't think Jesus would see it that way. African-Americans like me have to deal with racism all the time. That should make us more sensitive to what gay people contend with. We should be champions for others who are oppressed rather than part of the oppression. Female–National Baptist Church

An executive in one Protestant denomination shared in a focus group that curriculum materials in her denomination completely avoid dealing with the topic of gay rights or of how gay people are treated. "Even if we do think homosexuality is a sin," that person said, "we still should care about how homosexual people are treated by society. Discrimination is wrong."

Some of the teens who participated in the study have a parent who is involved in a homosexual relationship. We did not include a direct item about the sexual orientation of parents in the survey, but the written comments and interview comments of teens make it clear that such situations are not rare. Some of the teens with a parent who is openly gay feel awkwardness and a little embarrassment about it, but most indicated that they have come to accept the orientation. Here are some of the comments:

My parents got divorced four years ago because my mother came out as a lesbian. She still loved my father, but things weren't working that well between them. I was hurt and angry at first, but I've come to recognize that Mom can't help what she feels. She and Betty have a close relationship, and I spend every other week with them. It felt very strange at first, but now it feels as normal as being at Dad and Beth's. Some of my stupid friends at school don't understand, and sometimes I try to hide the fact that Mom is a lesbian. I feel like a traitor to her when I do that, but I want so much to be normal. Female–Mennonite Church

Dad is gay. Mom isn't. Both of them are in relationships with other people now. I stay at Mom's most of the time, but I can go to Dad's whenever I want. It's awkward when Dad and Ralph touch each other in front of other people. My friends think it's gross, and it causes me to be embarrassed about Dad . . . . I probably shouldn't feel that way, and I know it hurts him when I act like I don't want him coming to my track meets or school plays with Ralph. Male–Episcopal Church

I like to say that I have two moms now. Mom and Kathy have been living with each other for three years. I spend more time there than at Dad's. . . . A few of my friends had trouble accepting Mom living with Kathy, but if they couldn't get over it, I figured that they weren't really my friends anyway. If you don't accept my parents, then you aren't going to be part of my life. . . . Female–Evangelical Lutheran Church

When Dad came out as gay, it was almost a relief to me. I'd known he and Mom had troubles and couldn't figure out why. At times I thought it was my fault. Then I understood that it didn't have anything to do with me. . . . It's been a lot harder on my little brother and sister. They don't know what to say to their friends about Dad and Bob. In some ways it would have been better for Mom and Dad to have kept living with each other until my brother and sister were older. . . . But I probably wouldn't have wanted to do that if I were them either. Male–Roman Catholic Church

I'm okay with the fact that my father is gay. Sometimes I get nervous. Is it in the genes? I feel like I've got all the heterosexual drives and desires and everything, but could that change? I don't want to be gay because it makes life too hard. Dad lost his job and several friends and the respect of his parents. I couldn't stand to lose everything that he has. Male–Assembly of God

Most of the young people who wrote comments about having parents who were gay saw themselves as being heterosexual. These heterosexual young people seemed, on the whole, more accepting of their gay parents than some heterosexual parents were of gay sons or daughters. Some of the most painful comments which were shared with us came from teens with a homosexual or bisexual orientation who had experienced significant rejection by their parents. It appears from the comments, however, that the initial rejection or shock sometimes diminishes with the passage of time. That does not always happen. There are also some parents who show strong acceptance of teens with a non-heterosexual orientation. Consider these comments:

I will be very thankful when I graduate from high school and can go away to college. My parents both freaked when I told them I was lesbian. My mother got over it in time and has tried to understand me and be supportive. My father doesn't act like he'll ever get over it. He avoids talking to me all the time. We'll sit at the supper table, and I'll talk to Mom and she'll talk to Dad. He hasn't given me a hug in two years. I know that Mom keeps trying to get him to be more accepting,

*but it isn't working. It hurts me so much and makes me sorry
that I told them. I should at least have waited until I was out
of high school.* Female–Roman Catholic Church

*My parents were shocked when I told them I was gay.
Dad asked me like three or four times in a row if I was sure.
But even in the very first conversation, they told me that I
was their son no matter what happened and that nothing
I would ever do would make them love me less. They meant
it. I know this hasn't been easy for them, but they've never
been critical of me. Dad joined PFLAG [Parents, Families,
and Friends of Lesbians and Gays] and has become an
advocate for gay rights. . . . Mom has been reading books
about the Bible and trying to get our minister to consider
the possibility that he may not understand the Bible as well
as he thinks. Both my parents have been great.* Male–
Pentecostal Church

*I've caused this awful tension and conflict in my family by
coming out. If I had it to do over, I wouldn't. My little
sister doesn't understand everything, but she's always sweet
to all of us–she's the best person in my family. . . . My big
sister is in college, and she's been very understanding.
My father has been cool with it all along. But my brother
and my mother are disgusted with it. My mother says that
it's a sin, and she's made me talk to our pastor twice.
My brother is the way he is because he has all these friends
who are homophobic. I'm an embarrassment to him. . . .
Our pastor was actually better about it than my mother.
He says there's a difference between an orientation and
behavior and that you can't help your orientation. He keeps
urging me to pray for help and says that my orientation
could change. I don't think it will. But I didn't feel like he was
condemning me. . . . My parents fight about this. My big sister
and my mother fight about it. Sometimes I think it would be
better if I just disappeared. . . . A week doesn't go by without
my thinking about killing myself.* Male–Missouri Synod
Lutheran Church

*My parents are divorced and remarried, so I have like two
families. I first told my mom about two years ago that I
thought maybe I was bisexual. She was understanding and
very helpful to me. Then I told her husband too, and he was
like totally okay with it. I can talk with both of them about*

*anything, and that's helped me sort things out. . . . My
dad is another story. He and my stepmom haven't been able
to handle it. They would probably do better if I had just
told them that I was a lesbian. They could handle that better
than my being bi. But I still think bi is what I am. I spend
more and more time at my mom's house because it's safe
there. . . . I love my dad so much, and it hurts me so much
that he can't accept me as I am. It's like he thinks this is a
reflection on him or that the divorce caused it. The divorce
didn't have anything to do with it, and I don't think anybody
caused it. It's just how I'm wired.* Female–United Methodist
Church

A pastor in a large congregation said that their church had
helped form a local PFLAG partly because he knew there were at
least three families in the church dealing with issues of sexual
orientation of a son or daughter. He said that the supportiveness of that group has helped many people in his congregation
and in the community. He shared in a focus group that he still
isn't sure himself where he stands theologically on whether or
not homosexuality is a sin but that he's very sure that God cares
about and loves homosexual people. It felt very important to
him for the church to provide help and support to parents and
young people who are struggling with issues of homosexual
orientation and behavior.

A Challenge for the Church

Few issues are as potentially divisive in faith communities as
the matter of homosexual orientation and behavior. While some
denominations are clearly accepting and others clearly in
opposition to homosexuality and bisexuality as orientation
and/or behavior, there are many others which are in continuing
struggle over the issue. Official denominational positions are
not always representative of what clergy and laity within the
denominations believe, feel, and think. One of our observations
from having read such extensive comments from youth and
adults and having listened to so many people in interviews and
focus groups is that there are very few denominations in which
one can find true resolution or consensus surrounding the
topics of homosexuality and bisexuality.

As the authors of this book, we have no illusion that anything we say is going to cause a change in the beliefs of readers on these topics. Our intention is to be respectful of the diversity of viewpoints. There are, however, some very deep concerns which we have:

- It is very important for congregations to recognize that almost all have at least some youth who are struggling with issues of sexual orientation. As sermons are preached, classes taught, and youth discussions directed, clergy and other leaders need to recognize the high probability that some of the youth participating see themselves as having a non-heterosexual orientation. Not recognizing that reality means that many hurtful comments can be made and increases the probability that these youth will not seek help from their faith-based institution. *Further, nonhetero-sexual teens in our study were almost twice as likely as heterosexual teens to have seriously considered suicide.*

- Both parents and teens have a strong need for safe places that these issues can be discussed. Faith-based institutions have the potential to provide those opportunities. It's time to break the silence on this issue in our work with youth. Sexual orientation and related issues need to be openly discussed as part of the congregation's youth program.

- Persons in traditions which continue to feel that homosexuality and bisexuality are abnormal or sinful need to be careful that those issues do not assume more importance than they should. One Missouri Synod Lutheran pastor shared the observation that: "Homosexuality is not the unforgivable sin. Living in a time where people die of hunger, where children and spouses are abused, and where violence has become commonplace in society, we need to keep some perspective."

- Persons in traditions which are accepting of homo-sexuality as an orientation and a behavior have the opportunity for significant ministries not only to their own youth but also to youth in the community who struggle with these issues.

• Adult leaders in all faith-based institutions need to recognize that religious faith and congregational involvement are very important to the youth of non-heterosexual orientation who participated in this study. Whatever the congregation's theological position on these issues, these youth need to experience love and acceptance.

Chapter Seven
How Much Are Congregations Doing?

*Our parish does a reasonably good job teaching
teens what is prohibited. The Church's positions
on premarital sex, birth control, homosexuality, and
abortion are made clear. In the process, I'm afraid
our teens aren't helped to see sex as a good gift from
God. We do far too little to help them prepare for
healthy sexual relationships in marriage or for
eventual parenting themselves.*

Roman Catholic Priest

A Better Climate

Christian Community's president and one of the authors of this book, Steve Clapp, conducted a similar though smaller study of youth in congregations fifteen years ago. The clergy we have encountered in focus groups and who have responded to our surveys in the current study, while often not proactive in enabling sexuality education in their congregations, are more realistic in their recognition of the need for more to be done than fifteen years ago.

Of course those willing to complete a survey on the subject are likely among the more open clergy, but it is encouraging that 68% of them agreed with this statement: "I think it is possible for us [as a congregation] to do more than we currently are [in sexuality education], and I would like to make that a greater priority than it currently is." Twenty-four percent agreed that "it is possible for us [as a congregation] to do more than we currently are [in sexuality education], but I can't make that a priority right now." Only 8% said "I don't think it is realistic for us to do more than we currently are."

Virtually no clergy felt that what they were currently doing was enough–including those in congregations which offer fairly

comprehensive sexuality education. There is a general awareness that much more needs to be done, even though there is
understandable anxiety about how to proceed.

The teenagers who completed surveys for us and who shared
in focus groups almost all want more guidance and support from
their faith-based institutions than they are currently receiving.
They would like more help in relating their faith to decisions in
the areas of sexuality, dating, and marriage. Many of them are
frustrated by the combined failure of their parents and their
religious institutions to offer them practical help in this
important area of life. Almost none feel that the public or
parochial schools they attend are offering them all the
information they need in the area of sexuality. Those attending
Lutheran parochial schools were the most likely to receive
information about sexuality in the educational process, but they
longed for more opportunities to actually discuss the issues.
Consider these comments:

> *Our youth group advisor went on this big rant and rave
> about how corrupting the Internet is, about how dangerous
> it is for teens to be getting information about sex from the
> Net. He's been great to me, and I don't mean to put him
> down. But he's like all the other adults in not wanting
> to give us information and then being shocked that we
> get it from other places. Health and Daily Living classes
> in school don't begin to tell you what you need. Your
> parents sure don't, and the church sure doesn't. So where
> do you find things out? The Internet and television and
> your friends. Don't blame us for where we go when you
> don't tell us anything.* Female–United Methodist Church

> *Our pastor came to the youth group to meet with us when
> we were doing a two-part session on sex. He was terrified
> to be talking with us about the topic. I felt sorry for him.
> But all he had to say was that we should not do anything
> until we get married. He even talked like kissing and
> holding hands were the start of the slippery slope down
> to pregnancy and abortion and AIDS. That is not what
> I call helpful.* Male–Assemblies of God

In comparison to a review of religious sexuality curricula
which was conducted fifteen years ago, the materials which are
available today are, almost without exception, improved. There

are some denominations which offered almost nothing fifteen years ago which today have resources available. The new *Our Whole Lives* curriculum from the Unitarian Universalist Association and the United Church Board for Homeland Ministries is very comprehensive and carefully designed. The Missouri Synod Lutheran Church offers sexuality education materials consistent with their faith tradition for every age level from young children through adults. Abingdon Press, Group Publishing, Focus on the Family, and other religious publishing organizations offer resources which can be helpful, depending on one's own faith tradition and philosophy about sexuality education.

Those positive comments need to be qualified, however, in two ways. First, we experienced substantial difficulty arriving at a survey design and distribution process which was sufficiently acceptable to pastors in more conservative and fundamentalist congregations for them to be willing to cooperate in the study. They are aware of the need for more to be done in this area, but they are also fearful of directly confronting the topic; and the frankness of the survey was a problem to some. Second, while the curriculum materials are better than fifteen years ago, most resources still fail to meet the needs which exist. Here's what some denominational and organizational leaders had to say (names and affiliations are not given to protect confidentiality):

- *We've produced some better materials than we had before, but they've been written with the most conservative voices in our denomination in mind. The dominant question when these materials were reviewed was continually: "Will this offend anyone?" rather than "Does this meet the needs of young people?" We would have produced something very different if the second question had been the focus.*

- *Everything this organization produces is focused on telling teens how dangerous sex is and on scaring them away from early sexual activity. We push pledges for virginity, and we push abstinence. We actively discourage giving teens information that would prepare them for mature sexual relationships later in life or that would actually equip them to deal with temptation in the back seat of a car. They have to go to the Internet and their friends for that information. I've tried to work for a different*

*approach, but our funding base is very conservative, and
we aren't going to change.*

- *This denomination almost ended up stopping the publication
  of all our materials related to sexuality education. The
  materials already were schizophrenic on the subject of
  homosexuality, just like our denomination is. We finally
  managed to keep the materials in print, but they aren't
  being revised or updated.*

- *The Catholic Church does more today than it did twenty
  years ago. That's, in my opinion, primarily because of
  AIDS and concerns about abortion and homosexuality.
  What we are not doing is giving our youth any comprehensive understanding of how their faith should relate
  to sexuality. I am afraid that the result is that these teens
  will all grow up thinking the church believes sex is bad
  and dangerous.*

Almost all of the 28 denominational and parachurch execu-
tives with whom we visited wished that more were being done to
help congregations work effectively with teens in the area of
sexuality. And most felt that, at the national level, there was
very little that they could do in the present climate which has
denominations and nonprofit organizations concerned about
not alienating current and potential sources of funding. There is
a fear that those who are offended by efforts to do more
comprehensive sexuality education will stop providing financial
support. Denominational leaders also fear becoming the focus of
debates over the handling of issues like homosexuality and
abortion.

What Grade Would You Give?

Clergy, youth group advisors and teachers, and the youth
themselves are not in agreement on the kind of job their
congregations are doing in providing sexual information and on
preparing young people for marriage and parenting. We asked all
three groups to "grade" the work their congregation was
currently doing as excellent, good, fair, poor, or nothing. Here
are the average "grades" given by each of those groups:

	Clergy	**Advisors/Teachers**	**Youth**
Sexual information	Fair	Fair	Poor
Marriage	Fair	Good	Poor
Parenting	Good	Fair	Poor

Some clergy did share in written comments that they weren't directly involved in their church's work in these areas, often leaving that responsibility to an education commission, a youth council, or the adult teachers and advisors who work directly with the youth. Thus some of them may be assuming that more has been done than has actually happened. The adult advisors and teachers, however, are almost all working directly with the youth and are aware of what is and is not happening in these areas. It is clear that the youth do not see the quality of the help they are receiving in the same way as clergy and the other adults who work with them view that quality.

Our intention here is not to be critical of clergy and other adults who work with youth. It is very important, however, for us to be aware that youth do not assess the quality of the guidance they are receiving in the same way that adult leaders do. When we talked about these differences in perspective in groups with which the initial survey results were shared, we received some comments like these:

I honestly do not know how anyone could think our church is helping you prepare for dating or marriage. I know the pastors do premarital counseling for people who've set a wedding date, but we almost never talked about these things in youth group or Sunday school. Teen Female–American Baptist Church

I bet we're part of the problem. We thought we were doing a lot with the True Love Waits program and an emphasis on abstinence, but I'm sure our teens have all kinds of questions that we never address. Adult Advisor–Pentecostal Church

Many of the kids I know, who are all black like me and go to the same school, are going to be parents before they ever get a high school degree. But the church doesn't teach us how to avoid getting pregnant, and it sure doesn't teach us what it means to be a parent. . . . We have one class at school where they ask you to carry this like robot baby around and take care of it. That's a good activity to help you see the problems of being young and pregnant. But it doesn't do anything to help prepare you to be a good parent. If nobody is going to teach us parenting skills, somebody had better teach us birth control. Teen Female–National Baptist Church

I like to think that the curriculum used in Lutheran schools gives our youth what they need. As I've been listening to some of the rest of you talk tonight, I think we might be doing a little better job than some of you because we do offer instruction through our school. But what I hear the teens here saying tonight is that we aren't creating a climate where they feel comfortable raising questions. Pastor–Missouri Synod Lutheran Church

As we actually looked more specifically at what congregations were doing in this area, we increasingly began to realize, from our perspective, that the youth seemed to be more accurate in their assessment than the adults.   When asked to indicate the approach to sexuality education in their faith-based institution, here's how clergy responded:

14%   said the congregation offers a reasonably comprehensive approach to sexuality education.

49%   said the congregation offers a limited amount of information and/or discussion in existing classes or groups.

37%   said the congregation does almost nothing.

Just how comprehensive the sexuality education is even in those faith-based institutions which do offer it may be a matter for debate.   While 14% of clergy felt that reasonably comprehensive sexuality education was offered, not all the youth in their congregations reported receiving all the information generally considered to be a part of comprehensive sexuality education.   Fewer than 14% of all the youth responding indicated that they had received any significant information from their faith-based institutions on:

• Contraception
• Preventing sexually transmitted diseases
• Preventing AIDS

- Rape
- Homosexuality

Youth were most likely to have received information on HIV/AIDS as a social issue, on abstinence, on dating, and on sexual decision-making. Eighty-nine percent of youth felt, however, that the information on sexual decision-making they had received was not adequate.

HIV/AIDS appeared to be a somewhat frequent discussion topic for an occasional youth class or group, but teens did not often receive information on the prevention of HIV other than under the heading of abstinence. The discussions about AIDS seem to be more as a social problem about which Christians should care than as an actual condition that could potentially happen to young people in the church. When asked "Do you know everything you need to avoid getting AIDS?", only 8.5% indicated that they did.

Rape is not a popular topic for discussion in youth classes or groups. Only 6% of the youth surveyed have participated in a church or synagogue class or group discussion focused on the topic of rape and its prevention. Most of them are also not receiving that information in school or from their parents. Almost all the females who completed the survey indicated that they needed help in knowing how to prevent rape and that they needed greater assertiveness skills.

Even among the 8% of the youth who have received information on contraception from their faith-based institution, the content of that information was relatively limited. Very few youth were even aware of the existence of emergency contraception, which could be an important alternative for persons who have been raped. The contraceptive information which is shared generally focuses on the condom and oral contraceptives, with very little said about other approaches.

The vast majority of youth classes and groups appear to approach the topic of homosexuality from the perspective that no one in the class or group could possibly be homosexual. That same attitude is reflected in the curriculum materials of most denominations. Thus even in those faith-based institutions where discussions about homosexuality are encouraged, the youth in the group who may self-identify as homosexual or bisexual may hear that orientation condemned without any consideration to the possibility that someone in the group has or will have that orientation. Many also have or will have family members and friends with that orientation.

A Healthy, Positive View

The three categories again showed differing responses when asked to indicate agreement with this statement: "My congregation portrays sex in a healthy and positive way."

- 74% of clergy agreed
- 76% of youth advisors/teachers agreed
- 44% of youth agreed

Clearly youth do not recognize the view of sex presented or found in the congregation as being as positive as adult leaders think that it is. Here are some comments:

Our pastor and our teachers make me feel like sex is an ugly, dangerous thing. But if that's what it is, why would anyone want to do it? Male Teen–Southern Baptist Church

I know that the adults who work with us care about our well-being. They don't want us getting pregnant or getting AIDS. But the way they talk about sex is always emphasizing the negative. They say it's "God's good gift," but the way they talk about it doesn't make it sound good. Female Teen–Presbyterian Church USA

I have a news flash for the adults in our church. Sex is fun. Sex is good. Having sex doesn't make something awful happen to you. If sex is as bad as they act like it is, how did any of us kids ever get born? Male–Free Methodist Church

I think it is difficult to balance teaching youth that sex is a good gift from a loving God with the fact that we want to prevent premarital intercourse, pregnancy, abortion, and AIDS. It's easy to get so focused on the warnings we give youth that we fail to give them an accurate

picture of how wonderful sex is in marriage. Pastor–
Episcopal Church

*We've used True Love Waits and Focus on the Family
materials with our youth. I think the materials are very
good in terms of cautioning youth about sex and helping
them see the spiritual dimension to sexuality. But I'm
uncomfortable with the role that fear plays in those
materials. Are we really preparing youth for the healthy
sexual relationships that we want them to have in marriage?*
Adult Youth Advisor–United Methodist Church

Teaching youth about sexuality is not, of course, an easy
task. As shared in Chapter Three, we asked clergy and adult
youth leaders to indicate how they felt about teaching both
abstinence and comprehensive sexuality education. Comprehensive sexuality education, as defined for the purposes of the
survey, includes factual knowledge about the body and
sexuality, scriptural and theological background, relationship
issues, pregnancy and sexually transmitted disease prevention,
and guidance in decision-making. Virtually all professionals
who work with sexuality education also maintain that it should
include the teaching of abstinence. We intentionally made
abstinence its own category because we wanted to see how
survey respondents viewed abstinence in relationship to more
comprehensive approaches. Here's how the clergy and other
adult leaders responded:

4.2%   Agreed that faith-based institutions should teach
        comprehensive sexuality education to teenagers
        and did not check teaching abstinence

30.3%   Agreed that faith-based institutions should teach
        teenagers to abstain from sexual intercourse and
        did not check teaching comprehensive sexuality
        education

61.5%   Agreed that faith-based institutions should teach
        both comprehensive sexuality education and
        abstinence

4.0%   Agreed that all sexuality education should be in
        the home and not in the faith-based institution

Overall, 91.8% of the clergy and other adults participating in the study think that it's important to teach abstinence. The minority who did not agree that it was important to teach abstinence either felt that only comprehensive sexuality education should be taught or that no sexuality education of teens should happen in faith-based institutions. A substantial percentage, 61.5%, felt that both abstinence and comprehensive sexuality education should be taught by faith-based institutions. This result generated some heated debate in a couple of group settings where these results were shared.

Our conviction, based on the survey results, the focus groups, and discussion of the results in various settings, is that a focus on abstinence alone or on virginity pledges does not constitute an adequate approach to sexuality education in faith-based institutions. The promotion of abstinence needs to be a part of more comprehensive sexuality education, which in religious settings should include the relationship of spirituality to sexuality. The reasons for this conviction:

- Formal virginity pledges in our study did not correlate with higher or lower rates of sexual intercourse. We don't want to discourage such pledges, since the Peter Bearman and Hannah Brückner study suggests that they may have an impact on less congregationally active teens than those in our study (see page 61 in Chapter Three). But we feel that congregations should not rely exclusively on that strategy, especially since, among the teens in our study, the formal pledge had no greater impact than the encouragement of abstinence without a formal pledge.

- The subgroup of teens in our study who showed significantly lower rates of sexual intercourse shared a number of characteristics. The fact that they saw their congregations encouraging abstinence was only one of those characteristics. While not all of the congregations of this subgroup were offering comprehensive sexuality education, they certainly were including some elements of that, including the provision of information on how to make sexual decisions and on what the Scriptures say about sexuality.

- Our study shows that when congregations provide contraceptive information to teens, it does not result in teens being either more of less likely to have sexual intercourse–but it does make them less likely to become pregnant.

- In our faith-based institutions, we care both about those teens who choose to abstain from intercourse until they are married and about those teens who do not make that choice. The majority of the teens in our study, while viewing sexual intercourse as a serious step, were not committed to waiting until marriage. If we talk more about the issues and the faith, we may be able to increase the numbers willing to wait. Providing appropriate factual information will help protect the well-being of those who do not wait until marriage, and that factual information will result in better sexual experiences for those who do wait until marriage.

- The teens themselves want their congregations to do more to help them with sexual decision-making. That was true for teens who have had sexual intercourse and also for teens who have not. Since teens themselves are requesting more comprehensive sexuality education, congregations should respond positively.

Youth clearly expressed a desire not only for more help in sexual decision-making but also for more help in preparing for marriage and for parenting. Those expressions were especially strong among African American and Hispanic youth.

Many youth offered comments about their frustration with the lack of information and guidance they receive from their congregations and also from school and home. Some also expressed appreciation for help they had received in a congregational setting, but the comments of frustration were more frequent. For example:

You want to know what information we get on birth control and AIDS. I'll tell you something–adults in the church and every-where else don't want to give you any information about any-thing. You will think I am the most ignorant person on the planet, but I didn't know what was happening when I started

121

my period. I was having this panic attack over it in school, and a friend explained it to me. My mother told me she had intended to talk to me about it when I was younger, but she figured health and gym classes in school took care of it. Nobody takes care of it. You learn from your friends. You learn from television. You learn from magazines. You can learn some from the web. But you aren't going to learn it from the people who should tell you. Female Junior–United Methodist Church

My church has a one word answer for everything. For drinking, smoking, doing drugs, s - - - - - - -. It doesn't matter. Just say NO. That's the message. They love to print up these little pledge things and give them to you to sign. It was smoking and drinking in the seventh grade. Then they got around to drugs when I was a freshman. Then when I was a sophomore, it was sex. So we all sign these pledge things, and then they get collected and posted on a bulletin board, and we have this little prayer time about it. You have to sign–or everyone will want to know why your card isn't posted. We all know it doesn't mean a thing. Male Sophomore–American Baptist Church

We had this wonderful youth group advisor when I was a freshman and a sophomore. She was a home ec teacher in one of the high schools, and she knew that we weren't getting the information we needed in any classes at school. We spent two months on Sunday evening talking about sex. She gave us all kinds of information no other adult had, and she made us feel comfortable asking questions. She had the pastor come one Sunday night to talk about the Bible and sex. That was really interesting, and it was the first I discovered that the Bible actually has good things to say about sex. It helped all of us. I'm sorry for my younger sister that we have a different group advisor now, so she probably won't get the same information I did. Female Senior–Church of the Brethren

I thought I was pregnant two years ago. I didn't know who to turn to, but I remembered that our youth pastor always said we could talk to him about anything. I went to him, and he was so great. It turned out that I wasn't pregnant. THANK GOD! But the pastor helped me see myself differently than before. He helped me see the spiritual part of myself. He didn't put me down about having had sex. He just wanted me to see the big picture. And he wanted me to use birth control if I was going to keep doing it. I think that may have been the most important

*conversation in my life. And he like totally honored my privacy.
He never told anyone, and he never made me feel uncomfortable
about what I had told him.* Female Junior–Church of God

*I am really glad that you are doing this survey. Something
needs to be done to get churches to see that we need help with
this part of life. I suppose it's just as hard for girls as for guys
but maybe in different ways. For a guy, you've got to act like
you're cool and know what you need to know. You can't act
ignorant with a girl, and you don't want to have other guys
knowing that you are dumb as a turd about all this stuff. . . . I
kind of thought that having oral sex wasn't the same thing as
having sex. My girl friend felt that way. She was willing to
give me a blow job but not to go all the way. We didn't know
that you could get a disease from it. And I sure didn't know
at the time how many others had been in her mouth. Between
the two of us, we ended up giving a disease to a lot of people.
Talk about stupid. But why doesn't anyone tell you anything
except don't do it?* Male Senior–Episcopal Church

Needed Resources

There are significant areas of agreement on opportunities
which clergy, youth advisors and teachers, and the youth themselves would like to see. At least 88% percent of the youth, 86%
of the youth advisors and teachers, and 71% of the clergy
surveyed would like to see each of the following:

- Books or other resources which youth can use privately
  to learn more about dating, marriage, parenting,
  sexuality, and sexual decision-making.

- Class or group study and discussion on the same topics.

- Opportunities for classes on those topics which are open
  to young people who are not members of the congregation and strategies for reaching out to those youth.

- Programs to help teens be more assertive and avoid rape,
  sexual harassment, and sexual abuse.

123

As we shared earlier in the chapter, the available resources are, in our opinion, considerably better than when we did a similar study fifteen years ago. Yet only 27% of the clergy surveyed felt that the existing resources from their denominations do a good job providing youth with the help needed in these areas. Many noted that their denominations provide nothing at all. Most clergy who visited with us in focus groups and who wrote comments on the survey would like to see resources which did a better job meeting the multiple objectives of:

- Placing sexuality firmly in the context of spirituality.

- Providing teens with the factual information they need about sexuality.

- Helping teens understand how to build healthy, positive relationships.

- Helping teens learn how to make healthy decisions about sexuality.

- Helping teens be prepared for dating, marriage, and parenting.

The youth who participated in the focus group discussions were concerned that many resources which we had on display did not seem to present sexuality in a positive way. The focus of many resources is so much on discouraging youth from early sexual intercourse that an overall healthy, positive view of sexuality isn't always conveyed.

There are other kinds of needed resources and strategies. Clergy expressed significant interest in:

- Strategies which would help build congregational support for more sexuality education among youth in the church and in the community.

- Opportunities to work cooperatively with other local congregations in efforts at sexuality education. This does not necessarily mean shared classes but rather a shared emphasis, which would be easier to implement because neighboring congregations were also doing so.

- Programs and resources to help parents be more comfortable talking about sexuality with their children.

- Training opportunities for themselves, adult youth workers, and parents.

Eighty-nine percent of the youth would like to see an Internet website designed specifically for teens that addresses both sexuality and faith concerns. That was affirmed by 68% of the youth teachers and advisors and 49% of the clergy. The lower levels of enthusiasm for that option from youth teachers and advisors and from clergy appear to reflect more ambivalence about the Internet than youth have.

In the next chapter, we'll share some strategies that have proven effective with youth. Hopefully you'll discover some approaches which can help improve work in your own congregation.

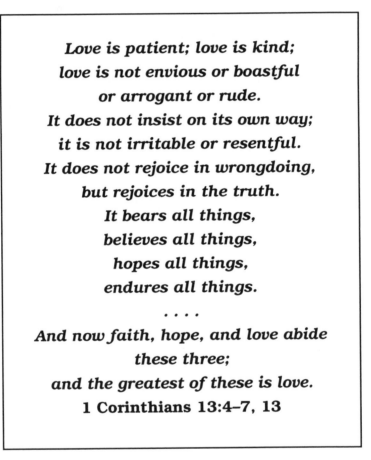

Love is patient; love is kind;
love is not envious or boastful
or arrogant or rude.
It does not insist on its own way;
it is not irritable or resentful.
It does not rejoice in wrongdoing,
but rejoices in the truth.
It bears all things,
believes all things,
hopes all things,
endures all things.

. . . .

And now faith, hope, and love abide
these three;
and the greatest of these is love.
1 Corinthians 13:4–7, 13

Chapter Eight
We Can Do More!

*What I got out of this that's most important is the
knowledge that I can help other people. There's so
much wrong information about sex. Now that I
know the facts and can relate sex to my faith, I
can also be a resource to my friends.*

Female, Sophomore
United Methodist Church

We Can Do More

As we have shared earlier in this book, congregations and religious organizations in the United States do seem to be at a point of greater interest in helping teens in the area of sexuality. Our own study found that, both in surveys and in focus groups, the teenagers themselves, clergy, and adult youth workers all want to see congregations doing more to help teens prepare for dating, sexual decision-making, marriage, and parenting. There are also other positive indicators including:

- The fact that the United Church of Christ and the Unitarian Universalist Church cooperated in the development of *Our Whole Lives*, which is a comprehensive sexuality education curriculum.

- The fact that the *True Love Waits* movement has gained momentum around the country with its emphasis on obtaining pledges from teens to abstain from intercourse until marriage. Some Catholic High Schools have "Chastity Days" which encourage abstinence.

- The Religious Coalition for Reproductive Rights has been actively at work encouraging African American churches to do more with sexuality education. They developed a curriculum called *Keeping It Real*, which we is being used in several black congregations.

- Many denominations offer resources in this area. The Missouri Synod Lutheran Church, for example, offers materials for all age levels from young children through adults.

- The National Campaign to Prevent Teen Pregnancy, which has been a high profile agency with excellent media contacts, has included faith-based emphases as part of its work.

- The Religious Institute on Sexual Morality, Justice, and Healing has been formed for the purpose of encouraging congregations to do more in this important area.

While the need for resources and strategies remains vast and we have significant development plans of our own, all the factors just shared are encouraging signs.

Since you've read this far in the book, our assumption is that you are interested in practical strategies which can help your own congregation or other congregations do more to help teens in these important areas. In this chapter, we are providing you with a some of the best strategies we've learned about through the study itself and our additional work with congregations, youth, clergy, and adult youth workers.

Factors to Incorporate

After the survey was complete, we met with groups of teens from diverse religious backgrounds at five different locations to seek their help in determining some of the factors that are most important in a congregation's efforts to be helpful in this area of need. Based on their input and on the results of the survey and the focus groups, we offer the following guidelines or factors to incorporate into congregational programs:

- Congregations need to clearly connect sexuality to spirituality. Teenagers need help in seeing themselves as the children of God and in relating their faith to sexual values and decisions. Congregations which design their programs primarily around resources from secular organizations need to be sure to incorporate an emphasis on religious faith.

- Congregations need to be sure that the resources used, the leaders who are involved, and the emphases made convey a positive view of sexuality rather than a negative view. With understandable concerns about early intercourse, teen pregnancy, AIDS, and other sexually transmitted diseases, it's no wonder that congregations so easily fall into emphasizing the negative. Youth, however, resent that tendency and also gain the impression that the congregation believes sex is something unpleasant or dirty. Don't let your approach become fear-based.

- Congregations need to teach abstinence to youth, but they also need to have sufficient confidence in youth to give them the factual information that they need to understand their own sexuality. As shared earlier in this book, teaching abstinence is important but youth also need factual information and decision-making skills.

- Congregations need to help youth be prepared for dating, including an understanding of the factors that are part of a healthy dating relationship. (Most youth also need help in understanding the factors that result in good, healthy friendships–with persons of either gender.)

- Congregations need to help youth be prepared for marriage and parenting. These are major life roles, and some congregations which do a good job providing information about sexuality do not follow through with the information teens need about marriage and parenting. The romantic concepts of marriage which are part of motion pictures, television, the Internet, and numerous magazines create unrealistic expectations of marriage and need to be put in perspective by congregations. Youth need to recognize that the characteristics which may attract them to another person are not necessarily the same characteristics needed in a lifetime partner.

- Congregations need to help youth develop healthy assertiveness rather than the too common submissiveness among young women and the too common aggression among young men. Healthy assertiveness protects youth not only in sexual situations but also in a large number of other life situations.

- Congregations need to help youth develop healthy decision-making skills, not only in relationship to sexual decisions but to other life decisions as well.

- Congregations need to recognize that how teens feel about and take care of their bodies relates strongly to the decisions they make about sexuality. It's important to help teens have the information they need about eating disorders, physical fitness, alcohol and other drugs, nutrition, and related concerns.

- Congregations need to offer help in the area of sexuality with an awareness that some of the teens will see themselves having a homosexual or bisexual orientation rather than a heterosexual orientation. While congregations which are opposed to homosexual behavior will need to present their position with integrity, that position should also be presented with an awareness that there will almost certainly be homosexual youth who are present. Congregations which can affirm homosexual orientation as well as heterosexual orientation can be important resources for youth in the community.

- Congregations need to equip their teenagers with knowledge not only for the sake of the youth themselves but also because educated youth can be valuable resources to other teenagers. With so many teens receiving their information about sex from the media and from their peers, teens who have the right information can be a great asset to other teens.

- Congregations should offer help to parents to enable them to be better sexuality educators for their own children and youth. Even congregations which are very uncomfortable with providing direct sexuality education to teens can equip the parents of teens with the information they need to help their own young people.

- Congregations which are not ready to offer all of the help suggested in the previous points should nevertheless work hard to do more than they currently are. Steps in the right direction make a difference.

Building Support in the Congregation

Obviously helping teens in the area of sexuality can be a controversial process in some congregations. There are a number of things which faith-based institutions can do to increase the willingness of adult members and constituents to help youth in this important area. For example:

- Pray about this need and encourage others to pray about it. God does work through the prayers of people, and prayers often help us put our fears into a healthier perspective.

- Start providing factual information about teens and sexuality in bulletins and newsletters. Refer to statistics and other information from this book. Help adults understand how much teens want help from the congregation in this important area.

- Provide factual information about teen pregnancy, HIV/AIDS, and other sexually transmitted diseases. While people need to come to an understanding of sexuality education as something that is concerned about more that problem prevention, the tragic statistics can often gain the initial attention of people. Share information about studies on teen sexual behavior that you find reported in local newspapers and other media in addition to information from this book.

- Provide copies of this book to those in the church who work with youth, to parents, and to members of the congregational board or other top decision-making group. The information will help people better understand why new actions need to be taken.

- Have speakers who are informed on the topic visit with classes and groups in the congregation. Invite a clergy person from another congregation which is doing more in this area to visit with leaders in your congregation.

- Have a study committee or task force formed with both youth and adults for the purpose of studying these concerns and making recommendations to the congregation.

- Teach a series of classes for adults based on this book.

- Encourage clergy to speak to these issues and concerns in sermons, meditations, and homilies. When clergy are behind initiatives, the chances of success are much greater. Sexuality should be related directly to religious faith, and clergy are the ones in most congregations with the strongest theological background.

- If your church has not been doing anything in this area, then your best starting place may be with a class or group for parents and for workers with youth. Then those persons will be better equipped to provide the help that youth need. This book can be a resource for such groups.

- Develop a plan to improve sexuality education and preparation for dating, marriage, and parenting over a period of time. It often isn't realistic to start all the new initiatives at once. For example:

  Year One: Have a series of classes for parents and and for adults who work with youth.

  Year Two: Begin having eight class or group sessions a year which help youth deal with various aspects of sexuality, dating, marriage, and parenting.

  Year Three: Begin offering truly comprehensive sexuality education for youth.

  Year Four: Begin offering comprehensive sexuality education for youth in the community who are not part of the life of your congregation.

  Year Five: Begin offering age-appropriate sexuality education to children and adults as well as youth.

- Work cooperatively with other congregations of your religious tradition or of other religious traditions to offer shared classes, groups, or other opportunities.

- Partner with secular organizations you trust to respect your faith-based perspective and who have experience helping youth in this area of need. Depending on your community and your theological perspective, this might include the YMCA, YWCA, Planned Parenthood, crisis pregnancy centers, Boys and Girls Clubs, and others.

Talking with Youth

As you read these pages, you may find yourselves wondering about your own comfort level in talking with youth about sexuality and related topics. You are not alone! Eighty-three percent of the clergy and adult youth workers who responded to our survey indicated that they need greater comfort and skill in talking with youth about sexuality. Here are a few suggestions and guidelines that may be helpful to you and to others in your congregation:

- Talk about sexuality and religious faith with other adults to gain more comfort handling the topic. Study groups with parents and other adults can be very helpful in that process. Discussion of the chapters in this book can make a difference for you.

- Decide how much you as a parent or other adult working with youth want to share about your own sexual values and experiences. It is NOT necessary to reveal everything you've done–and that could well be embarrassing to you and your teenagers. On the other hand, your own willingness to talk about temptations, difficult decision-making, or your own lack of knowledge in the past may create greater openness on the part of your young people. Teens respect the candor and the honesty of adults.

- Use statistics like those in this book and information on secular studies from the news media to initiate discussions with teens. It's easier to talk about statistics or what other people have said than to talk about personal experiences. Ask: Do you think that many teens in your school do this kind of thing? Are you surprised by these numbers? What do you think about this information?

- Motion pictures, television shows, and the Internet can all provide openings for discussion. Ask youth for their opinions about the way sex is portrayed in a motion picture. Ask how they feel about advertisements that use sex as a motivator for sales. Go to motion pictures and watch television shows that you know your young people are viewing. You'll be much better prepared to relate to them.

- Talk plainly and be nonjudgmental about contraception and other questions teens may raise about sex. Don't assume that because a teen is interested in talking about contraception that he or she is already having sex. Such questions are appropriate ones for young people to be raising, and you should be pleased to be part of a conversation about the topic.

- Don't assume that teens have all the information they need. As earlier chapters have made clear, teens have a great deal of misinformation about sex. They need your help in having the right information.

- You may need to do some personal reading and study to be sure that you have the right information to share with teens in the congregation. Many adults in our focus groups talked about not having current information on newer kinds of contraception and about not knowing the facts on HIV and other sexually transmitted diseases.

- When one of the authors of this book was in seminary, the "common wisdom" was that children and youth should have their questions abut sex answered but shouldn't be given any more information than they are requesting. That is probably bad advice for today. As quickly as young people are finding themselves in situations that require knowledge about sex, they need to have solid information from us. Try giving them more than they ask for!

- Listen to teens! That means allowing them to fully express themselves before adding comments. Try to avoid showing shock or surprise over what they say; focus your own mind on being thankful that they are talking frankly with you. Accept the right of teens to have their own feelings and opinions, no matter how unorthodox or controversial they may seem to you to be. You shouldn't express agreement that you don't feel, but your being respectful of their opinions will make it much more likely that they will be respectful of yours.

- Use "I" language in talking about your own values, beliefs, and opinions. Don't get trapped lecturing with "you" statements which may seem accusatory to a young person.

- Remember that youth learn from what we do as well as from what we say. When parents treat each other and their children with respect and courtesy, that example conveys a great deal to their children about how persons should relate to each other. Most people primarily learn about parenting and about how married persons treat each other through observation. None of us are perfect, but many of us can work at improving the example we set.

- Be sure that your conversations about sex are not continually focused on prohibitions. Sexuality is a good gift from a loving God. Convey that to the youth who are part of your life at home or in the congregation.

- Youth who are connected to a congregation and who have other meaningful community involvements are less likely to have early intercourse than youth who are not so connected. Encourage youth to have high levels of congregational activity, to be involved in the community, and to do things to help others. These activities will enrich their lives in many ways.

- Be sensitive to how concerned most teens are about their appearance and about the appearance of their friends. If youth who are in your home or in your congregation clearly want to improve their physical

135

appearance, help them find healthy, appropriate ways to do so. Good nutrition and regular exercise can improve the appearance and the overall health of most of us. At the same time, however, most youth need help understanding that human worth is something much deeper than outer appearance. Teach youth and model in your own life that the worth of a person is not synonymous with appearance. Teens who select dates and friends heavily on the basis of appearance are setting themselves up for frustration and for lost opportunities. That is also the path to disastrous marriage choices for many people.

• Parents who want more help talking about sexuality with their teens can find excellent guidance in Debra Haffner's book *Beyond the Big Talk: Every Parent's Guide to Raising Sexually Healthy Teens–From Middle School to High School and Beyond* [Newmarket Press, 2001]. The book contains a great forward by her daughter.

Strategies for Work with Youth

Some congregations are already offering comprehensive sexuality education, and the authors of this book hope that your congregation is part of that group or becomes part of that group. You may well feel, however, that comprehensive sexuality education would be much too great a step for your church at the present time. You don't have to start there, and suggestions about other strategies have been offered at other places in this book. Gathered here are some options to consider:

• As already discussed in this chapter, offer training for parents and for the adults who work with youth.

• If you aren't ready to offer formal training for those adults, you can help simply by making copies of this book and other resources available to them.

• Provide reading materials for youth which can help them relate their faith to sexuality and which offer them the factual information that they need. That could include materials available from your denomination, copies of this book, or appropriate resources from community agencies. See the *Resources* listing at the end of this book.

- Use motion pictures to generate discussion on these topics. *A Walk to Remember* raises issues of abstinence. *Cruel Intentions* is a movie for mature audiences but raises many serious issues about sexuality and about how males and females treat each other. Movies can quickly become dated, but sexual themes are so pervasive that there will almost always be reasonably current videos, DVDs, or theater films that raise important issues.

- Use this book itself as a resource for a series of classes or group discussions with teens. The next chapter gives suggestions for several sessions built around the chapters you have been reading.

- Use a topical approach to this area through existing youth classes and groups. Have discussions on topics like:

  - Your Body and Your Faith. How do teens feel about their bodies and the bodies of others? How can they have healthier lives? How do they feel about the emphasis which our society puts on physical appearance? What does the Bible teach about the body?

  - Decision-Making 101. What are the factors that should be a part of decision-making about sexuality or any other issue? How does our religious faith influence our decision-making?

  - Dating 101. What factors are involved in deciding to ask another person out? What are the differences between the factors that attract us to others and the factors that make for long-lasting relationships? How should people treat one another when dating? How should religious faith influence the way we treat others in the dating process?

  - What Do You Know about Sex? Have an anonymous quiz on sexuality to find out what youth in your class or group know. Share and discuss the results, correcting misinformation in the process. Include some questions about the teachings of your faith-based institution regarding sexuality.

- Have a session focused on positive reasons for waiting before having intercourse. Encourage honest and open discussion about the reasons people have early intercourse, and involve the teens themselves in generating reasons for waiting. Relate the discussion directly to the teachings of your faith tradition.

- Have a session on alcohol and drugs and in the process talk about their influence on sexual decision-making. How should our faith affect our use of alcohol and drugs?

- Have a session on male and female roles. Talk about the changing roles of men and women in our society. How do youth feel about male and female roles? What roles do males and females have in dating relationships? In what ways are these roles healthy or unhealthy? Talk about the role religious faith has played in the development of those roles. What changes do young people think need to be made in those roles?

- Have a session on sexual orientation. What are the factors that cause people to be homosexual, heterosexual, bisexual, or transgendered? In preparation for the session, give youth opportunity to write their questions and concerns on notecards. Talk about the way that homosexual persons are treated in our society. What does our religious faith teach about sexual orientation? About the way that all persons should be treated?

- Have a session which deals with HIV and other sexually transmitted diseases. Include a factual quiz as part of the session to be sure young people have accurate knowledge. Try not to let the session become fear-based. Talk about societal attitudes toward persons who have AIDS and discuss how congregations should respond to such persons.

- Have a session on healthy assertiveness and rape prevention. Help teens understand the differences among submissiveness, aggressiveness, and assertiveness. Relate healthy assertiveness to religious teachings about respect for persons.

- Have a session focused on ways that the media influence our views of our bodies and of sex. Tape selected advertisements and clips from television programs that are relevant. Talk about these relative to religious faith.

Some people may be comfortable creating their own sessions from the brief sketches just given. You can likely find resources from your denomination which deal with at least some of the topics. There are study materials from *Group Publishing* which deal with some of the topics. You can also use *Faith Matters* as a resource for some of the sessions. See the *Resources* section at the end of this book for some suggestions.

A Report on a Local Emphasis

The authors of this book have wanted to identify practical ways that the information from this study on teens, sexuality, and religion could be utilized to the benefit of local congregations and communities. With help from The Lutheran Foundation, we decided to undertake a pilot project in our hometown of Fort Wayne, Indiana. From a political perspective, Fort Wayne is generally considered a conservative community, though it is possible for Democrats to be elected mayor and congressional representative. Fort Wayne is sometimes known as the "City of Churches" and does have a large number of strong congregations including Roman Catholic, mainline Protestant, and evangelical churches. Both the Missouri Synod Lutheran and the Evangelical Lutheran denominations are especially prominent in the community. Fort Wayne also has moderately good diversity for a Midwestern city of its size. In addition to the black and Hispanic populations, there are large numbers of Vietnamese and Burmese. A Burmese Buddhist Temple is located just a block away from the Anabaptist congregation in which one of the authors of this book worships.

The pilot project was titled "The Ties that Bind." The title was chosen because of the gospel song "Bless'd Be the Tie that Binds," which talks about the binding together of hearts in love. Our goals in the project included:

* Making clergy and other leaders in local congregations aware of the results of our study and of the implications for their important work with youth.

* Getting at least thirty congregations to take some new initiatives in helping teens be better prepared for dating, marriage, sexual decision-making, and parenting.

* Getting at least a few congregations to take some initiatives in reaching out to youth in the community.

We made no effort to persuade congregations to accept a particular theological perspective or to use a particular set of resources. Wherever possible, we made congregations aware of the resources which already existed within their faith tradition. Our intention was to be respectful of the particular theological heritage of each congregation but to make clergy and other leaders more aware of the importance of helping teens relate their faith to their sexual decisions.

Our efforts were somewhat handicapped by the fact that many denominations do not have current resources in this area of need and that the quality of some of the resources which are available is not always high. The interactions with local congregations deepened our own awareness of the need for more resources to help teens relate their faith to decisions about dating, marriage, sexuality, and parenting. We were in each instance, however, able to find a way to help congregations improve their work in this area.

In our planning for this emphasis, we underestimated the extent to which churches and pastors have to be at a point of "readiness" to take this kind of action. We also underestimated how much staff time would be needed to set up and keep appointments with clergy and other church leaders. While we had direct contact with pastors or other church leaders in 171 congregations, there were another 148 congregations with which we had no substantial communication beyond the mailings which we sent to them. We have been pleasantly surprised, however, to discover that those written communications actually continue to produce results months after the official end of the program. We are still receiving calls from congregations which are now at a point in time at which they are interested in doing more in this area.

We ended up with thirty-five congregations which took some kind of new program initiative, and there are another nineteen congregations considering such an initiative as this book goes to press. Overall, we were very pleased with this result. The new initiatives varied considerably, ranging from hosting a seminar for parents to help them become better sexuality educators to training youth to be accurate sources of information to other teens in the community.

For the most part, we intentionally did not work with local media on this project. We felt that congregations were more likely to participate if their involvement was low profile. One of the coauthors of this book, Steve Clapp, was invited to speak on this topic to a Forum at Indiana-Purdue University Fort Wayne, and the videotape of that presentation was broadcast perhaps twenty times over the University's cable station. That exposure did generate several calls for additional information about the program.

We were pleased to find considerable receptivity to our efforts on the part of some community agencies which are essentially secular in focus. These agencies nevertheless recognize that the moral and spiritual dimensions of decisions about sexuality are important. The Boys and Girls Club and Whitington Homes and Services, a local agency especially focused on the needs of pregnant teens, have cooperated with us and plan to do more with us in the future. There are other community organizations with which we made contact and which have indicated an openness to further cooperative work–including Big Brothers, Big Sisters; the Center for Nonviolence; the Girl Scouts; and the YWCA.

As part of this project, we decided to do a local study which utilized the same format as our national survey. We encountered clergy and other leaders in Fort Wayne who found it difficult to accept the possibility that youth in their congregations were likely to exhibit the same values and behaviors which we had found in our national study. Although a few Fort Wayne area congregations were part of the national study, those did not represent a large percent of the total. We decided that it was important to do a new local study so that we would have Fort Wayne regional data which could readily be compared with the national data. What we found was that the values and behaviors of church-active teens in the Fort Wayne area were essentially the same as the national study had shown. This data has been very helpful in persuading local clergy that steps need to be taken at improving help to youth, and the data has also been of interest to secular youth-serving organizations in the community.

As we sought to customize our services to meet the needs of particular congregations which were interested, we developed some new models of workshops for adult youth workers and parents. In response to requests from many pastors and other adult youth workers, we developed an extensive listing and description of resources in this area.

We are very much aware, however, that the thirty-five congregations which have participated with us in the Ties that Bind program represent only a little more than ten percent of the congregations in the Fort Wayne area. We recognize that a tremendous need exists for continued initiatives to be taken in helping congregations do more to empower their youth with the information they need. Many of the congregations which did not participate in the Ties that Bind program will at a future time be ready for new initiatives if the training, resourcing, and consciousness-raising takes place. We have plans for future work in this area in our own community.

We hoped from the conception of the Ties that Bind program that this might become a model for other communities and organizations. Regional denominational judicatories (synods, districts, conferences, presbyteries, regions, and dioceses) and secular agencies which are wanting to more fully involve congregations in sexuality education should consider taking the proactive step of visiting with clergy throughout the geographical area. The fact that we went directly to clergy rather than asking them to seek us out made a great difference. We would encourage other communities considering such an emphasis to:

- Anticipate that making connections and visiting with clergy and other leaders is a very lengthy process and that congregations and clergy must be at a point of "readiness" to have interest in such visits.

- Concentrate primarily on workshops and training that take place in individual congregations rather than on community wide events.

- Take initiatives to encourage training events and other resourcing for parents of youth and for adults who work with youth. Congregations which are very nervous about any kind of sexuality education can often be persuaded to take an initiative to better prepare parents and adult youth workers to help teens.

Teach me, O Lord,
the way of your statutes,
and I will observe it to the end.
Give me understanding,
that I may keep your law
and observe it with my whole heart.
Lead me in the path
of your commandments,
for I delight in it.
Turn my heart to your decrees,
and not to selfish gain.

. . . .

Teach me good judgment and knowledge,
for I believe in your commandments.

. . . .

Your word is a lamp to my feet
and a light to my path.
Psalm 119:33–36, 66, 105

Chapter Nine
Sexuality and Spirituality:
Empowerment for Young People

*Reading what other teens think is a tremendous help
to me. It makes it easier for me to get clear about my
own beliefs. I can't wait to see the book with the full
results. The way people at school talk makes you
think everyone is having sex. It's a big help to know
that there are others who aren't ready and that there
are others who think God should be part of your
decisions.*

Male, Junior
Presbyterian Church, USA

A Study Guide

This chapter is essentially a study guide for individuals and
groups wanting to think more deeply about the issues raised in
Faith Matters. While some secular organizations may share in
study of this book, our anticipation is that most groups which
gather for discussion of these pages will be in congregational
settings. This guide will be most useful for those in Protestant,
Roman Catholic, or Jewish settings; but we hope that persons of
other faith traditions will find at least some of the suggestions
helpful.

This guide does anticipate the possibility that it may be
studied by youth classes and by youth groups as well as by
adults. The quotation which begins the chapter comes from a
teenager who was in one of the early groups in which some of
the results of the study were shared. He and the other teens
who have seen the data and heard or read the comments of
people their own age have shared a desire to see the entire report
and to talk about it. If your congregation has not been doing
much with sexuality education, the book you are holding could
be a starting point.

The suggested discussion questions and other activities are organized to follow the chapter divisions in the book. If you are doing this with a class or group, you may in some instances want to devote more than one session to a chapter. Individuals using this guide may want to record their responses to questions in a spiral-bound notebook or journal. Some of the activities are clearly more appropriate for use by groups than by individuals. Here are a few suggestions if you are doing this study with a class or group:

- Remember that every group has both active and passive learners. Encourage, but do not force, participation. Allow "I pass" as an acceptable response.
- Having class members use different translations of the Bible will enrich your discussion and give new perspective. Jewish groups using this resource will probably choose to disregard the New Testament references.
- Sessions assume, for groups, that a chalkboard or flip chart is available.
- While your sessions will be smoother if group members read the chapters in advance, it's not generally wise to assume that all have done so! Provide summaries to help those who have not read the material and to refresh those who have.
- We recommend that you open and close sessions with prayer.

Questions and Activities for Chapter One
Religion, Teens, and Sex–A Fresh Look

1. Read the opening quote. How do you feel about what this teenager says? *I know what I did is my responsibility, but the right information could have changed my life.* What is your congregation currently doing to help young people with dating, marriage, sexuality, and parenting? What else is needed? What are the barriers to doing more?

2. Look at the two definitions of sexuality on page 13, one from James Nelson and the other from the Surgeon General. Which definition do you like best? Why? What is positive about these definitions? How do these differ from the statement which follows? *Sex is something dirty and unpleasant. Save it for the one you love.*

3. **Primarily for teens.** Complete the *What Do You Know?* exercise which begins on the next page. Then talk together about the items and identify areas in which the group would especially like to have more information or more opportunity for discussion. No one should be pressured to share his or her individual responses to the items. One possibility is for the leader to photocopy the exercise onto plain paper for everyone in the group, let people complete the forms without putting their names on them, collect the forms, and then shuffle them and redistribute them for discussion. That way the responses to which you refer for discussion are those of someone else.

4. Look at the observations of teens on congregational life which are on pages 24, 25, and 26. Which ones do you identify with most strongly? Why? In what ways does the church at its best help young people? All people?

5. Assign the Old and New Testament readings which appear on page 28 to members of the group. Have each person look up one or more passages and then share with the group how the passage relates to the topic of sexuality.

Questions and Activities for Chapter Two
Sexuality Is More than Sex
(Material for at least two sessions)

1. **Primarily for teens (but also good for adults).** Give each member of the group an index card or small slip of paper. Have each person write one of the following on the card to describe how he or she feels about his or her body (you may wish to put these options on chalkboard or a flip chart):
  • Definitely unhappy
  • Somewhat unhappy
  • Happy but want improvement
  • Happy
Collect the cards, shuffle them, and then put tallies of the responses on chalkboard or newsprint. Note that in the study reported in *Faith Matters*, 61.9% of females were somewhat or definitely unhappy with their bodies, and 19.5% were happy but wanted improvement. Do those figures surprise you? Why, or why not? Why is physical appearance so important in our society? What's wrong with placing too much emphasis on physical appearance?

147

What Do You Know?

*The items which follow are concerned with the amount of knowledge and background which you feel you have in the area of sexuality, dating, and marriage. Mark an **X** on the line following each item to show how characteristic that item is of you. **7** indicates "very characteristic" and **1** indicates "not at all characteristic."*

1. I understand what all these words or phrases mean: erection, penis, vagina, labia, clitoris, orgasm, masturbation, ejaculation, HIV, sexually transmitted diseases, climax, oral sex, hymen, Norplant, sexual intercourse.

7	6	5	4	3	2	1

2. I have a good understanding of what happens during male and female sexual response. I understand what causes sexual arousal; why men often climax before women; and what the nature of orgasm is.

7	6	5	4	3	2	1

3. I can talk about sexuality comfortably with one or more friends. I do not feel embarrassed in talking about sexual concerns and can be honest about my own anxieties.

7	6	5	4	3	2	1

4. On a date, I can comfortably (or feel that I could comfortably) talk with the person I am dating about my own sexual desires and limits. I could listen to and respect the desires and limits of the other person.

7	6	5	4	3	2	1

5. I understand what the Bible and my faith tradition say about sexuality, and I know how to relate my faith to sexual decisions.

7	6	5	4	3	2	1

6. I know what characteristics are important to me in a marriage partner. I have worked through in my own mind the difference between the characteristics which attract me to someone and the characteristics which I would value in a marital relationship.

7	6	5	4	3	2	1

7. I feel secure in my own sexual orientation, and I understand at least some of the reasons why not all persons have a heterosexual orientation.

7	6	5	4	3	2	1

8. I am clear about my own values in the area of sexuality. I know under what circumstances I am personally willing to take part in sexual activities.

7	6	5	4	3	2	1

9. I understand the contributions to my sexual values which have been made by my parents, friends, school, congregation, television, magazines, and the Internet. I know how to comfortably sort through conflicting information.

7	6	5	4	3	2	1

9. I have a good understanding of contraception and know how to protect myself and a partner against both pregnancy and sexually transmitted disease.

7	6	5	4	3	2	1

10. I am always respectful of myself and of others as the children of God.

7	6	5	4	3	2	1

2. Page 32 has a comment from a young woman who had a birthmark on her face which was surgically repaired. She says, *When I had the ugly blotch on my face, it was easy to know who cared about the real me, the me that no one sees on the surface.* How do you feel about what she says? What role do advertisements, television programs, motion pictures, and the Internet have in shaping the importance we place on physical appearance? How can you better see the "real me" in yourself and in others?

3. Look on page 36 at the characteristics of those youth who had the lowest rate of sexual intercourse reported in the study. Which of those characteristics would be easy for youth to develop in your congregation? Which would be difficult to develop?

4. Look on page 37 at the differences in rates of sexual intercourse for the congregationally involved teens in this study in comparison to what secular studies have found. Do you think it is possible that teens who are having sexual intercourse may be less likely to be involved in the life of a congregation? Why, or why not?

5. Look at the section on oral sex on pages 41 through 43, including the statistics and the comments from teens. Are you surprised by the numbers of teens having oral sex? Why, or why not? Why do some people choose it instead of sexual intercourse? What concerns do you have about teens who are having oral sex?

6. Look at the section titled "Are Premarital Intercourse and Oral Sex 'Wrong'?" which begins on page 43. Why do you think there are such differences between what teens see their faith communities believing and what they personally believe on these topics? Do you think the views of teens on these topics would change if there were more open discussions in the faith community? With which of the comments from teens do you most agree? Why?

7. Look at the section on "Kissing, Petting, Being Naked" which begins on page 48. Are you surprised by the percentages of teens who have done these things? Why, or why not? Why do you think the authors of this book put these statistics after the data on sexual intercourse and oral sex rather than before? This

section also talks about dry humping. How do you feel about
that activity? How different do you think petting is from oral sex
or sexual intercourse–just a matter of degree, or is the difference
greater? Why?

8. Look at the statistics and comments about masturbation
which are on pages 52 and 53. Do those figures surprise you?
What, if anything, does your faith tradition teach about
masturbation? In spite of the fact that the majority of teens
masturbate, this is a very uncomfortable topic for
conversation–why?

10. Page 54 lists twelve "Sexuality and Spirituality–Guidelines for
Religious People." These were developed with the interaction of
youth in five different congregational settings. Go through the
guidelines carefully. With which ones do you most strongly
agree? Why? Are there any of them with which you disagree?
What guidelines would you add?

11. Look at the creation story in the first and second chapters of
Genesis. What do these words say about the goodness of
creation? How is that goodness reflected in the gift of sexuality?

Questions and Activities for Chapter Three
Abstinence

1. This chapter talks about abstinence as a positive choice
more than as a prohibition. Look at the comments from teens
on pages 55 and 56. With which of those comments do you
most strongly identify? How do those teens feel about the choice
not to have sexual intercourse? List on chalkboard or a flip
chart all the reasons your group can identify in favor of
abstinence and all the reasons for not emphasizing abstinence.

2. Look at the section on "Abstinence and Comprehensive
Sexuality Education" which begins on page 57. Why are most
clergy and other adult leaders more comfortable teaching
abstinence only than teaching comprehensive sexuality
education? What appear to be some of the shortcomings of
teaching abstinence only?

3. How do you feel about the pledges which programs like True Love Waits ask teens to take? See the discussion which begins on page 60. What are some of the positive benefits of such pledges? Why don't the pledges seem to make a greater difference to teens who are active in a faith-based institution? What impact happens to teens who make such a pledge and then break it?

4. Beginning on page 64, the authors of *Faith Matters* argue that it is important for abstinence to be a part of comprehensive sexuality education rather than the only approach used by a congregation. What are their reasons for that position? Do you agree or disagree? Why? Some people have suggested that the only reason for not providing full information about sexuality to teens is that adults do not trust them. Do you agree with that statement? Why, or why not?

5. In 1 Corinthians 3:16–17 and 6:12–20, Paul talks about the body as God's temple. What significance does that image have for discussions about sexuality? What significance does that image have for the way we take care of our personal health?

Questions and Activities for Chapter Four
Contraception

1. **Primarily for teens (but also good for adults).** Give each person a notecard, have them number from one to seven, and then have them write TRUE or FALSE in response to the following statements:
    (1) The pill protects against HIV and other STDs.
    (2) A woman can get a shot every three months that offers protection against pregnancy.
    (3) Condoms fail too often to be worth using.
    (4) If you put a condom on incorrectly or use the wrong kind of lubricant with it, the condom will not be effective.
    (5) There is no emergency contraception or "morning after" pill or pills that can prevent pregnancy.
    (6) The pill isn't very effective in preventing pregnancy.
    (7) The pill often has side effects that are fairly serious.
Collect the cards, shuffle them, and redistribute them. Then do a tally of the responses on chalkboard or a flip chart, having group members read off the response of the card they hold rather than their own. The correct answers can be found on pages 74

and 75. If everyone read the chapter before your class or group session, you'll have perfect responses! Ask whether or not any of this information was new to people in the group. Why is it so important to have accurate information on these topics?

2. **Primarily for teens.** Page 76 describes an activity which one youth group did in which people sat across from someone of the opposite sex, maintained eye contact, and then spoke aloud words having to do with sexuality. Do this exercise. If you don't have an even number of males and females, then you can use some same sex pairings for the exercise. Words to try: clitoris, vagina, penis, labia, condom, pill, arousal, orgasm, ejaculation, erection, climax. Then talk about how people felt about doing the exercise. Why is it important to be able to use these words in communication? What does it say about our society that we are so often uncomfortable talking about sexuality?

3. Look at the quotes on pages 69 and 70 about different ways that people handled pregnancy. How do you feel about their decisions? How could these situations have been avoided? Why is it important for people to be aware of the reality of God's forgiveness and acceptance, no matter what they've done?

4. Why does abortion emerge as an attractive option for many who have an unwanted pregnancy? Were you surprised to find that 50% of the teens who became pregnant decided to have an abortion? Why, or why not? What could their congregations have done to help them avoid becoming pregnant? What could their congregations have done to create a climate in which they would have felt they could have given birth to a child?

5. Read John 2:1–11 in which Jesus blesses the wedding at Cana by changing water into wine. What does this passage suggest about the importance of marriage? What does the fact that Jesus changed the water to wine say about the place of pleasure in our lives?

6. Do married couples have advantages over single parents in raising children? Why, or why not? Why do unplanned pregnancies create so many pressures and difficult decisions? What is the difference between a pregnancy being unplanned and unwanted?

Questions and Activities for Chapter Five
Unwanted Sexual Experiences

1. **Primarily for teens.** Distribute notecards and have people number from one through five. Then have them respond YES or NO to each of the following statements:
    (1) I know someone who has been raped.
    (2) I have had an unwanted sexual experience.
    (3) I feel assertive enough to keep from doing something sexually that I don't want to do unless physically forced.
    (4) I need better communication skills for talking with a partner or potential partner about sexual decisions.
    (5) I need help becoming a more assertive person.
Collect, the cards, shuffle them, redistribute them, and then tally the results on chalkboard or a flip chart. Are you surprised by any of the results? Why? Why do you think unwanted sexual experiences happen to so many people in our society?

2. Talk about differences between males and females in terms of having unwanted sexual experiences and communicating clearly about what they do and do not want to do. Page 82 has a quote from a parent about male and female roles where sex is concerned. Do you agree or disagree with the quote?

3. Page 92 lists some guidelines for "Equal Dating." In what ways can equal dating make it less likely that people will have unwanted sexual experiences? How do you feel about the guidelines which are given? What guidelines would you add?

4. Look at the differences in the statistics on page 83 between the unwanted sexual experiences which males and females have had. Why are those differences so large? How do you feel about the fact that only about half of the girls who have had unwanted sexual intercourse feel that it was rape? Do you agree or disagree with the reasons given on page 84? What role does communication play in avoiding such experiences? What role does healthy assertiveness play?

5. Pages 87 through 90 talk about "Unwanted Sexual Experiences with Adults." What could have been done to prevent some of the experiences which are described in this section? What needs to be done to help those who have been victims of such experiences? How do you feel about the story of the stepbrother and stepsister who shared in sexual activities?

6. Read 2 Samuel 11 and 12 which tell the story of David and Bathsheba. Do you think David used physical force when he first committed adultery with Bathsheba? Why, or why not? Why would it have been difficult for Bathsheba to be completely free to accept or reject David's advances? What are the consequences which come from David having Uriah killed? What evidence is there that God eventually forgave David for what he had done?

Questions and Activities for Chapter Six
Gay, Lesbian, and Bisexual Youth

1. **Primarily for teens.** Distribute notecards and have people number from one through five. Then have them respond YES or NO to each of the following statements:
    (1) I have friends who have a non-heterosexual orientation.
    (2) A gay or lesbian person can find welcome and acceptance in our congregation.
    (3) A gay or lesbian person can be open about his or her orientation in our youth group.
    (4) My congregation teaches that homosexuality is a sin.
    (5) I do not think that people choose a particular sexual orientation; they just "are" what they are.
Collect, the cards, shuffle them, redistribute them, and then tally the results on chalkboard or a flip chart. Are you surprised by any of the results? Why?

2. Look on page 96 at the percentages of teens with non-heterosexual orientations. Are you surprised by these figures? Why, or why not? The development of sexual orientation is one of the tasks of the adolescent years; to what extent do you think that may be reflected in these percentages? What are the implications of these percentages for church programming?

3. This chapter talks about the reality that most teens of non-heterosexual orientation have not been open with clergy or other adult leaders about that orientation. Why aren't they more open? Does your congregation offer an atmosphere in which teens with a homosexual or bisexual orientation would be comfortable talking about it? What could be done to improve the atmosphere? Why is it important for teens to be able to discuss their orientation in religious settings?

4. Pages 101 through 103 discuss the importance which teens of non-heterosexual orientation place on their faith and their involvement with a congregation. What kinds of struggles do youth have when their orientation is homosexual and the congregation does not approve of that orientation? Why do you think these teens continue to be involved in the congregation? Will that involvement change as they move into the young adult years? Why, or why not?

5. Read the story of the Good Samaritan in Luke 10:25–37. What does this parable suggest about whom we are called to love? What are the implications of this parable for the manner in which congregations relate to persons of homosexual or bisexual orientation?

6. Pages 108 through 110 offers "A Challenge for the Church." How do you feel about the suggestions made by the authors? Which are things your church is already doing? Which suggestions are possibilities for your congregation? Which are not likely to happen? What other suggestions would you offer to congregations for work with gay, lesbian, bisexual, and trans-gendered teens?

Questions and Activities for Chapter Seven
How Much Are Congregations Doing?
(Probably more for adults than for youth)

1. Why is the topic of sexuality such a difficult one for our congregations? What controversies about sexuality exist at the national level in your denomination? How ready is your congregation to do more to help youth relate their faith to their sexuality?

2. Page 115 shares the "grades" which youth, adult teachers and advisors, and clergy give to their congregation's work on helping youth with sexual information, marriage preparation, and parenting preparation. Why do you think the grades given by youth are so much lower than those from the adults? What do you think the grades would be for your congregation?

3. Pages 116 and 117 list several topics which are recommended as part of comprehensive sexuality education in faith-based communities. Which of those are covered by youth classes or

programs in your congregation? Which need to be covered? Which appear to you the most difficult to cover?

4. Pages 121 through 123 include several comments from youth about the help they have received or not received from their congregations. With which comments do you most strongly identify? Which comments would be most true for your congregation? What concerns do these comments raise for you?

5. Read 1 Corinthians 13, which is one of the most familiar passages in the New Testament. What do these words about love suggest for the congregation's work with youth in the area of sexuality?

Questions and Activities for Chapter Eight
We Can Do More!
(Probably more for adults than for youth)

1. Pages 128 through 131 list several factors which the authors feel should be incorporated in a congregation's efforts to help youth in the areas of sexuality, dating, and marriage preparation. Which factors are already incorporated into your congregation's program? Which factors need to be incorporated? Are there any factors with which you disagree? Why, or why not? Are there any factors which you would like to add?

2. The next section in the chapter, pages 131 through 133, gives several suggestions for building support in the congregation for more efforts to help youth in these areas of need. Which two suggestions would be the most effective in your congregation? What steps can you take to implement those suggestions? What additional ideas do you have?

3. **Primarily for adults.** Pages 133 through 136 provide very specific guidelines or suggestions to help adults talk with youth about the topic of sexuality. Go through the guidelines carefully. Are there any with which you disagree? If so, why? Are there additional guidelines you would like to add? Which are the ones which speak most strongly to you?

Primarily for teens. If teens are discussing this chapter, look at the guidelines on pages 133 through 136 and determine which ones apply to *you* in terms of conversations with your parents and other adults. What additional guidelines would be helpful to teenagers in trying to communicate with adults about sexuality?

4. Look at the strategies for work with youth which begin on page 136. Make decisions about the most appropriate strategies for your congregation at this point in time, and then begin planning to implement those strategies.

5. Read Psalm 119:33–36, 66, and 105. These verses talk about loving God's law and commandments. Why do you think the psalmist had such a positive view of the laws and rules of God? What is the purpose of the laws which we find in the Bible? What are the implications of these verses for relating spirituality to sexuality? Is the overall message of Scripture one of legalism or one of love? Why?

Resources

Organizations

Christian Community. That's the organization responsible for the book that you hold in your hands. Christian Community focuses on research and resource development to benefit congregations and the communities in which they minister. In addition to research and development on teens and sexuality, the organization has also developed resources on faith-sharing, hospitality, worship, and stewardship. 6404 S. Calhoun Street, Fort Wayne, Indiana 46807. 800-774-3360. DadofTia@aol.com; www.churchstuff.com

The Center for the Prevention of Sexual and Domestic Violence. This organization works with faith-based institutions to address sexual and domestic violence. They offer books, videos, and seminars. They can refer victims to sources of counseling in a local area. 2400 N. 45th Street, Suite 10, Seattle, Washington 98103. 206-634-1903. www.cpsdv.org

The Black Church Initiative. This is a project of the Religious Coalition for Reproductive Choice and has the goal of breaking the silence about sexuality in African-American churches. They have sexuality education curricula for both adults and teens, and they hold an annual National Black Religious Summit on Sexuality. 1025 Vermont Avenue, N.W., Suite 1130, Washington, DC. www.rcrc.org

The Religious Institute for Sexual Morality, Justice, and Healing. This is an ecumenical, interfaith organization dedicated to advocating for sexual health, education, and justice in faith communities and society. They offer resources, consulting, and seminars to help congregations become sexually healthy faith communities. 304 Main Avenue, #335, Norwalk, Connecticut 06851. 203-840-1148. www.religiousinstitute.org

National Campaign to Prevent Teen Pregnancy. This organization brings together people from many different fields in cooperative efforts to prevent teen pregnancy. They offer a wide range of resources, including some developed especially for faith-based institutions. They have a website packed with helpful information. 1776 Massachusetts Avenue, N.W., #200, Washington, DC 20036. 202-478-8518. www.teenpregnancy.org

The Center for Sexuality and Religion. This organization focuses on the education of clergy in the area of sexuality and works in cooperation with seminaries. 987 Old Eagle School Road, Suite 719, Wayne, Pennsylvania 19087-1708. 610-995-0341. www.CTRSR.org

Group Publishing. This is a nondenominational organization which provides a variety of resources for Christian congregations including some which deal with sexuality. P.O. Box 481, Loveland, Colorado 80539. 1-800-447-1070. www.grouppublishing.com

Publications

Drill, Esther, Heather McDonald, and Rebecca Odes, *Deal with It!: A Whole New Approach to Your Body, Brain, and Life as a Gurl.* Pocket Books, New York, 1999. Warning: This is a completely secular publication but contains a tremendous amount of information which can help adults who want to better understand youth and sexuality.

Haffner, Debra W., *Beyond the Big Talk: Every Parent's Guide to Raising Sexually Healthy Teens–From Middle School to High School and Beyond.* Newmarket Press, New York, 2001.

Haffner, Debra W., *A Time to Build: Creating Sexually Healthy Faith Communities.* The Religious Institute, Norwalk, 2002. (See the address on the previous page)

Kirby, Douglas, *No Easy Answers: Research Findings on Programs to Reduce Teen Pregnancy.* The National Campaign to Prevent Teen Pregnancy, Washington, DC, 1997. (See the address on the previous page)

Moore, Kristin Anderson, Anne K. Driscoll, and Laura Duberstein Lindberg, *A Statistical Portrait of Adolescent Sex, Contraception, and Childbearing.* The National Campaign to Prevent Teen Pregnancy, Washington, DC, 1998. (See the address on the previous page)

Nelson, James B., *Body Theology.* Westminster/John Knox Press, Louisville, 1992.

Sexuality and the Sacred: Sources for Theological Reflection, edited by James B. Nelson and Sandra P. Longfellow. Westminster/John Knox Press, Louisville, 1994.

Whitehead, Barbara Dafoe, Brian L. Wilcox, and Sharon Scales Rostosky, *Keeping the Faith: The Role of Religion and Faith Communities in Preventing Teen Pregnancy.* The National Campaign to Prevent Teen Pregnancy, Washington, DC, 2001. (See the address on the previous page)

Christian Community is in the process of establishing a Teen Empowerment Center which will link people to religious resources to help teens in the area of sexuality and which will develop new resources in this area of need. Beginning in the fall of 2003, we will offer an occasional print and online newsletter called **The Teen Empowerment Idea Kit**, *which will be available without charge. For more copies of* **Faith Matters**, *for a subscription to the newsletter, for questions about resources to help teenagers, or for information on our other resources, feel free to contact us at DadofTia@aol.com or 1-800-774-3360.*